THE 3

THE 3

How to Shred Fat, Get Healthy, and Be Fit Without Counting Calories, Calculating Macros, or Starving—and Keep Eating the Delicious Food You Love

STEVE HOCHMAN

Published by Best Seller Publishing®, St. Augustine, FL
Best Seller Publishing® is a registered trademark.
Printed in the United States of America.
ISBN: 978-1-969338-09-0

This publication is designed to provide accurate and authoritative information with regard to the subject matter covered. It is sold with the understanding that the publisher is not engaged in rendering legal, accounting, or other professional advice. If legal advice or other expert assistance is required, the services of a competent professional should be sought. The opinions expressed by the author in this book are not endorsed by Best Seller Publishing® and are the sole responsibility of the author rendering the opinion.

For more information, please write:
Best Seller Publishing®
1775 US-1 #1070
St. Augustine, FL 32084
or call 1 (626) 765-9750
Visit us online at: www.BestSellerPublishing.org

Disclaimer

I'm not a doctor. I'm not a registered dietitian. I'm not a licensed nutritionist. I'm just a guy who weighed 287 pounds 25 years ago, figured out a system that worked, and helped thousands of people transform their bodies.

That said, this book is for informational purposes only. Nothing in this book should be considered medical advice, nor should it be used as a substitute for professional medical guidance. Before starting any fitness, nutrition, or exercise program, you should consult your physician or a qualified healthcare provider—even if most doctors don't know jack about nutrition.

By using the information in this book, you acknowledge and accept that you are doing so at your own risk. The author and publisher disclaim any and all liability for injuries, health conditions, or other outcomes that may result from following the content in this book.

If you want a dietitian to put you in a calorie deficit and make you miserable, go for it. But don't say I didn't warn you.

Praise for Steve and *The 3*

From Stuck to Stronger Than Ever

Before working with Steve, I was exhausted, in constant stomach pain, and lost after cutting dairy. I'd tried every diet, but nothing worked. Steve didn't just give me a plan—he taught me how to eat for *my* body. I now have more energy, no pain, and real confidence in my nutrition. This experience has been life-changing.

— Lori

Found My Fire Again

I'd been in a funk for years, and Steve's program was the blessing I needed. He's genuine, kind, and the community he's built inspires me daily. I finally understand nutrition—without feeling like I'm dieting. This is just the beginning. Let's go! 🔥

— Mariel

Twenty Pounds Down at 57!

After years with OC|FIT, I still wasn't seeing the change I wanted—until the 28-Day Fat Shred. I lost nearly 20 pounds, learned how to eat right, and now people stop me to ask about my arms. I've kept the weight off and feel stronger than ever. I'm 57 and thriving!

— Dina

From Dad Bod to Six-Pack

I've been with Steve for over a year, and the results speak for themselves—hello, six-pack! The accountability, nutrition guidance, and weekly check-ins made it all possible. This program was simple, effective, and life-changing.

— Matt

A Mindset Shift That Changed Everything

This isn't just another diet—it's a complete mindset shift. I've let go of obsessing over food, built lean muscle, and kept the weight off. Steve's program transformed my body—and elevated my life.

— Laura

Better Than Before Baby

After having a child, I felt stuck. Macros, keto, long workouts—nothing worked. Steve gave me a new perspective, immediate results, and better fitness than I had before pregnancy. It was truly transformational.

— Cleydi

No More High Blood Pressure or Kidney Disease

At 57, I'm in the best shape of my life. With Steve's help, I reversed my high blood pressure and early-stage kidney disease—through nutrition alone. I love how I feel, and I'm forever grateful.

— Mike

Discipline I Needed, Results I Wanted

Steve keeps you accountable and informed—answering every question and reading every food log. His healthy swaps and focus on clean eating helped me stay on track and see real results. Abs are made in the kitchen!

— Amber

No More Diet Struggles—Just Results

After years of failed weight-loss attempts, Steve's 3-Rule program finally worked. I never felt restricted, hit my weight goals, and now have the confidence to tackle anything. Empowering and transformative.

— Natalie

A Coach Who Truly Cares

Steve patiently taught me how the body works and how to fuel it properly. I dropped weight, lost inches, and gained muscle— all without starving or counting calories. His support and the weekly coaching calls made all the difference.

— Steve

Stronger, Leaner, and Healthier

After a lifetime of struggling with weight, this program changed everything. The 3 Rules work. I've reshaped my body, healed my relationship with food, and feel healthier inside and out.

— Grace

Fitness and Food That Changed My Life

I thought I was just getting old—until Steve showed me how simple lasting change can be. His nutrition plan and workout program transformed my body and boosted my endurance, especially on my last ski trip. I feel incredible.

— Hillary

Dedication

This book is dedicated to my first mentor, Travis Mayfield, the man who taught me the true meaning of mental toughness, how to set goals, and why the words *can't* and *try* have no place in my vocabulary.

Your belief in me and your mentorship didn't just guide me—it changed the entire course of my life.

Great leaders don't just inspire with their words; they lead through their actions. And you did exactly that.

You will always be my mentor, my adopted father, and the person who made all the difference.

Table of Contents

**Chapter 2: Rule 1—Stay Below 25 on
the Glycemic Index** **57**

Acknowledgments

I didn't do this alone—far from it. This book exists because of the incredible people who supported, guided, and believed in me along the way. I owe them more than words can express, but this is my best attempt.

Thank you to my best friend and wife, Stefanie, whose belief in me makes me feel like I can accomplish anything. You are my rock, my heart, and my greatest blessing. I couldn't have done this without you.

To my kids—Kayla, Riley, and RJ—you are my driving force, my bigger purpose. Everything I do is with you in mind, and I hope this book serves as proof that you can chase your dreams and make them real.

To my mom—through my lowest lows and highest highs, your love and support have never wavered.

A huge thank you to Best Seller Publishing, specifically my writing coach, Cat Lauria, for your guidance, patience, and expertise in bringing this vision to life. Your support made all the difference.

And to everyone who has ever believed in me, challenged me, or pushed me to be better—thank you. This book is as much yours as it is mine.

What Is The 3?

The 3 is a way of being as lean, fit, and healthy as possible without feeding a host of diseases while enjoying the foods that you absolutely love. You never have to be calorie restricted, starving, or carry around a calculator so you can count your macros at every meal.

Once you understand the ingredients in your food, specifically the hidden ingredients that are causing massive fat storage, it's simply a matter of deleting or replacing one or two ingredients of your favorite foods. Now you can enjoy all the food that you used to feel guilty about cheating with. When you understand The 3, you understand how ingredients work, and by making slight changes in the way you eat, you can have it all.

The 3 Rules are simple and will cut through all the deceptive food industry's BS, exposing the hidden ingredients that are causing you to store fat. You will literally be shocked when you learn what foods and ingredients, many of them considered "health foods," are doing to your body.

Rule 1: Here, you will master the glycemic index (GI). Once you understand this concept, getting lean for the rest of your life is pretty easy.

Rule 2: You'll focus on which foods, when combined, cause you to store fat and how you can avoid those combinations.

Rule 3: In "Strategic Carb Timing," you'll learn the best and *most effective* time to have carbs to get lean and strong.

After that, I'm going to show you my three accelerators. The accelerators are used to amplify the results of "The 3."

Accelerator #1 is the Magic Fat-Shred Drink, which is a delicious formula that not only hydrates you but curbs hunger, helps you manage cravings, and burns fat.

Accelerator #2 is my Magic 36-Hour Fast. I'll teach you how to burn 2 to 3 pounds of pure fat in 36 hours without feeling hungry!

Accelerator #3 is Intermittent Fasting. A lot of people are doing intermittent fasting *wrong,* and most people actually gain fat by breaking their fast incorrectly. I'll teach you how to accelerate your results by intermittent fasting at an expert level.

You might wonder why this is necessary. Why do you need to know every ingredient in your food? Why do you need a system like The 3 to follow, when technology is getting better and better every day? Shouldn't there be some easy way to make everything work for you?

Sure, technology is improving. Our understanding of health and fitness is increasing. But so are obesity, diabetes, heart disease, and cancer. In fact, these diseases are skyrocketing; but why?

Here's the real problem: Scientists in the food industry create ultra-processed ingredients and chemicals to get you addicted and leave you unsatiated to maximize their profits at your expense. They're not intentionally making you fat, but one of the most powerful components of their business model is using super-addictive ingredients in their products, which is why you gain so much weight.

Just think, with all this technology and health advancement, we as a nation should be getting healthier. But check out the mind-blowing statistics over the past 75 years from the 1950s to now.[1,2]

Obesity: 6% → 65%
Overweight: 22% → 78%
Heart Disease: 3 → 50 (per 10,000 individuals)
Cancer: 2 → 35 (per 10,000 individuals)
Diabetes: 1 → 45 (per 10,000 individuals)

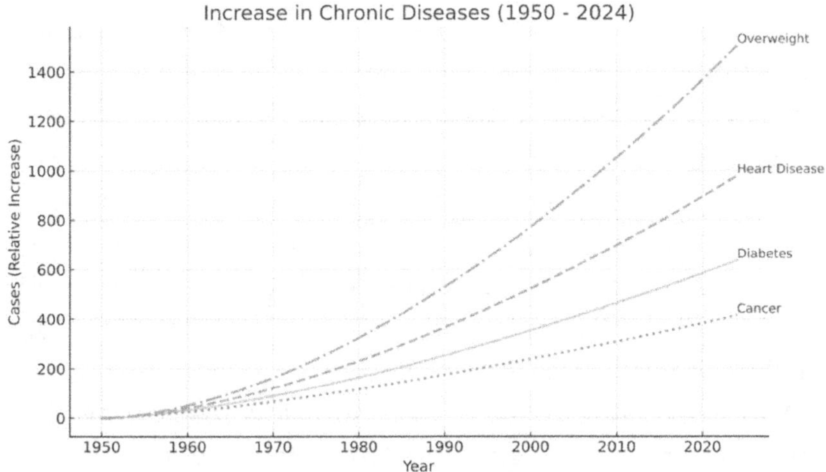

Technology *did* get better, *a lot better*. But unfortunately, it got better for the food industry, and now they are able to make even *more powerfully* addictive, ultra-processed ingredients. At the speed with which obesity and diabetes is increasing, soon nearly everyone will be obese and more than half of us will suffer from diabetes, not to mention a host of other diseases that feed off glucose. There is no question: *we are at war* with

---

1   Hales, C. M., Fryar, C. D., Carroll, M. D., & Ogden, C. L. (2017). Prevalence
    of Obesity Among Adults and Youth: United States, 2015–2016 (NCHS
    Data Brief No. 288). National Center for Health Statistics.
2   USAFacts. (2023, March 21). US obesity rates have tripled over the last 60 years. Retrieved
    from https://usafacts.org/articles/obesity-rate-nearly-triples-united-states-over-last-50-years/

the smoke and mirrors and deception of the big food industry, whose only goal is to make more profits.

The problem with that is that their profit comes at your expense. And the problem with *that* is that these ultra-processed, addictive ingredients and chemicals also release massive amounts of glucose, which then causes obesity to skyrocket, along with diabetes, heart disease, cancer, and many other diseases.

The food industry has you beautifully, strategically distracted with calories. The reason why is because the last thing they want you to do is look at the real problem, which is ingredients. Focusing on the calories is actually to their benefit because a lot of their offerings are 100 calorie, portion-controlled foods. In reality, they're charging you more per ounce for their "healthy alternative." They're giving you less and making more, all while keeping you distracted from learning the real root cause of so many health issues. This distraction is a huge problem.

You know what I'm talking about. How many times have you started to lose weight, or *actually* lost weight, only to find yourself completely miserable, plateauing, and starving? Not only are you not able to maintain it, but when you finally give up and go back to the way you were eating before, you're worse off because now you've decimated your metabolism by barely eating anything *and* you've lost muscle. Now, eating the same amount as you did before has an even worse effect. You're gaining more weight.

You go through the cycle over and over again, only to throw your hands up in despair because you know that slowly killing yourself through starvation is not sustainable, and it's not the answer. Nothing feels right about it.

It gets worse. If you're a parent, deep down, you know that you're passing your pain on to your kids because you haven't found a solution. You can't tell your kids "What you need to do is starve yourself, and that's how you're going to get leaner and be healthy." Let's be honest, *you* can't even starve yourself like that because it makes you miserable. And bonus! It's actually going to be worse for your kids because food scientists are getting even better at making more powerfully addictive foods that dump more glucose into their bloodstream. That's why you're seeing childhood diabetes skyrocket as well. So not only are you passing your pain on to your kids, you're passing it on with an exponential bonus.

You also know you're not giving your spouse the best version of yourself. To truly love someone is to give them the best of you. But you don't know how to do that because every time you've tried, you've failed. At this point you're like "I can either starve and be miserable, or I can be happy and just accept my unhealthy self and give my spouse this version of me because I don't know what else to do."

The whole game is rigged, but The 3 is going to free you from all this bullshit. When you look at everything through the lens of The 3, these big corporate food companies won't be able to fool you anymore because what they try to sell you won't make it through your new filter. We're going to shut down this excess glucose production. We're going to eliminate the ingredients that are making you unhealthy, but we're *not* going to make you resort to cheat meals to have your favorite chocolate lava cake. We're going to make it so that it actually makes you lean, fit, and healthy by using the correct ingredients. Not only is this the best solution, it's the only solution.

Are you ready? *Let's go*!

GIFT PAGE

I want to thank you more than you know.

Because with each transformation …

Each parent who now passes health down to their kids …

Each person who breaks free from their vices and regret …

It gives me the gift of living a life of purpose.

So in the spirit of reciprocity, I want to give you a *gift*.

Go to **SteveHochman.com** and use code **231407A** to get **lifetime access** to my entire digital library of **3 Rule–Approved Fat-Shred** recipes—delicious, easy-to-make, and designed to keep you on track.

And with **a new recipe added every week**, you'll always have fresh, fat-shredding meals at your fingertips.

This is my way of saying thank you for being part of this movement.

Let's transform together. Let's go!

Where It All Began

Somehow, this book ended up in your hands. Either through a friend, Instagram, a podcast, a bookstore, or divine intervention. No matter how it happened, you are now holding the *real* answer. The answer that I wish I had when I was nearly 300 pounds with dangerously high blood pressure and massive anxiety. The answer to how to be *lean, healthy,* and *happy* without counting calories, calculating a single macro, or starving yourself.

After reading this book, you will know without any doubt that The 3 is the *only* simple, sustainable, and effective way to end the weight gain epidemic. Bold statement? Keep reading.

The *problem* is that the whole game is rigged. Literally rigged. Without The 3, there is no way for you to be *lean* and *healthy* without practically *starving*. This is because everyone is focused on the *wrong* thing—calories. And the big food industry wants to keep it that way because it skyrockets their profits at *your* expense. They don't want you to *focus* or even *know* about the ultra-processed *hidden* ingredients they are intentionally putting in your food to keep you *addicted* to their products. The side effects of these ingredients directly result in steady weight gain while feeding a host of metabolic diseases like diabetes and heart disease. Babies, kids, and adults are unknowingly consuming hundreds of them on a regular basis. How else is it that as technology and access to information gets exponentially greater, we are getting exponentially fatter and unhealthier at the same time?

You've tried and failed at everything (counting calories, carb cycling, keto, paleo, not eating past 6 p.m., carnivore, intermittent fasting). Maybe you had some temporary success, only to go right back to where you were—or worse. Practically everyone has experienced the yo-yo effect. And because nothing has worked, millions of people are now desperately turning to a *lifetime subscription* of the pharmaceutical industry's dangerous drugs as a "solution." (Yeah, as if that's going to work out!)

People are sick, people are unhealthy, people are embarrassed about or not proud of the bodies we're given to live our life in, and I want to change that. This book is going to make it so you never have to count calories, you don't have to weigh your food, and you don't have to starve yourself. This book will show you the path to being lean and healthy for the rest of your life.

How? By the time you finish this book, it'll be obvious what's been missing in your life this whole time. By following the 3 Rules, you're going to know how to take charge of your life and solve your problems once and for all.

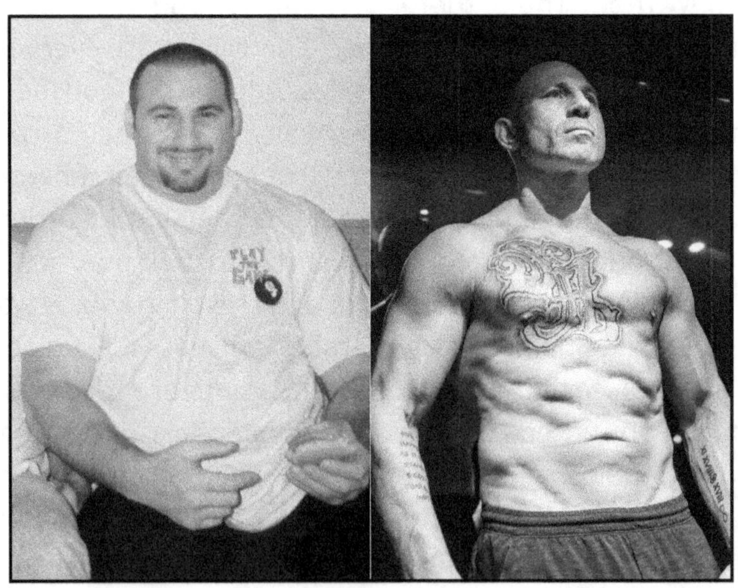

The photo on the left is me before The 3, when I was 22 years old. I was obese, had dangerously high blood pressure, and massive anxiety. The photo on the right is me after The 3 at 50 years old: confident, purpose-driven, and with a six-pack most guys half my age don't have. I've already helped thousands of people change their lives for the better, and I'm going to help millions, starting with you.

I didn't start at the top—hell, I didn't even come up from the middle of the pack. I scraped my way up from some of the lowest places a person can be. The message of this book is "If I can do it, you can too." I truly believe that, and I think it's important for you to know where I came from so you can understand how I got to where I am today. I wasn't born with the genetics to be lean easily, I've been homeless twice, and the first half of my life was an uphill battle. So, when I say "If I can do it, you can too," I really mean it.

I was born in Encino, California, in 1974. When I look back on my childhood, I don't have very many happy memories. My early life was filled with pain, frustration, and a lot of anger.

As a little boy, I had the sense that something was wrong with me. When I was five years old, I was diagnosed with Tourette's syndrome. My symptoms included shaking my head, saying unexpected words, and making noises and uncontrollable movements. If someone put something fragile in my hand, I had the irresistible impulse to crush it. If I was given a glass to drink from, I would often bite it until it broke. The feeling of needing to move or vocalize to get relief would build up in me until it burst out, over and over. That was my everyday existence, and it was horrible.

The only thing that gave me any temporary relief was a focus on extreme physical exercise. Baseball was my first sport, and I would go to the batting cage and hit ball after ball. It wasn't until junior high school that I started to grow out of it a bit, and by the time I hit puberty, the symptoms had mostly faded away.

Despite my symptoms improving, socially, I was still an outcast. Lunch was always stressful because I didn't have a group of people who wanted me around. People tended to avoid me, like they could feel that something was off. I'm not sure if it was just because I didn't have much practice, or part of my condition made me unable to intuitively know how to "fit in," but one way or another, I ended up by myself most of the time.

Outside of school, I played baseball. I was a catcher. I was pretty good, too. I even got noticed by a scout from the Minnesota Twins organization. Stats don't lie, and with my batting average and performance behind the plate, I made the All-Star Team. But because of my underdeveloped social skills, I was benched most of the time. I was just the kid who had something "off."

It was a different story in school, where I never got picked for any sport. I took my rage out in two-hand touch football in PE, launching people off their feet for not choosing me for their team. That's when another kid said to me, "Why do you play a sissy sport like baseball? In football, you can literally try to destroy people, and you won't even get in trouble." That was all I needed to hear.

In tenth grade, I walked onto the football field to try out for the team. I didn't show up for football to play football. I showed up because I had so much anger and frustration that I just needed to hit people—I didn't care if it was a teammate, if it was practice, or during a game. If we won, fine, I didn't care—I just needed to release all the *rage* and *anger* that I had built up inside.

Meanwhile, at home, things were in constant chaos. Every few months, my father and I would move to a different apartment or house. I didn't know at the time that the reason for this was because my dad didn't have a real job. He told me he was an "insurance consultant," but in actuality, he was a con artist who was always trying to scam people out of money. He would blame our getting evicted from our homes on the "postal service." Every check he was expecting got "lost in the mail."

Eventually, we got kicked out of our last house. We had no place to go, so we lived out of a car.

At the end of my first year playing football in the tenth grade, I decided I was going to get a football scholarship. I had no logical reason to believe I could do it, but I was *positive* that I could. A scholarship was going to be my way out of living in the car.

I went to my football coach and told him that my goal was to get a scholarship. He laughed and told me that it was impossible. He said that I had only played one season and was competing with guys who had been playing their entire lives. On top of that, he told me that I wasn't that good at football; I was just aggressive.

I said, "Watch me." I was going to be the one in ten thousand players who made it.

Despite all my father's terrible traits, the best thing he ever did was brainwash me into believing that I could do *anything*. He told me that I would be the best football player in the country, and I truly believed the man who, at the time, was my hero.

My whole life became *working out*. My father had me running sprints for hours, and he'd stand outside Gold's Gym smoking a cigarette and watching me lift weights through the window. He somehow even got me coaching on speed and explosiveness from Los Angeles Raiders player Stefon Adams.

In my senior year of high school, I was required to attend a special education class. I was embarrassed by it, but one day my teacher asked us to write down our top five goals. I *definitely* knew my goals, so I wrote them down.

STEVE HOCHMAN'S GOALS

Get a full scholarship to the #1 ranked football school in the nation.

Get a full scholarship to the #2 ranked football school in the nation.

Get a full scholarship to the #3 ranked football school in the nation.

Get a full scholarship to the #4 ranked football school in the nation.

Get a full scholarship to the #5 ranked football school in the nation.

I was *dead serious*. The teacher kept me after class and told me to aim lower, for something I could actually achieve. He said junior college would be "more realistic." There was an awkward moment when I stared at him. I stood up, and at 6'3" and 240 pounds, I towered over him. He turned pale. At the time, I'd never seen a grown man do that. No more words needed to be said.

It was time to get mine. I was *obsessed*. Most of the high school football players did just the minimum in lifting weights with the team. I did the team workouts plus my own. The other players hit with pads only with the team, at practice. I "borrowed" pads and a helmet from the equipment shed and drilled full contact all summer with my friend Albert and his teammates, who played junior college ball. Albert was a beast and one of my few friends. He would even let me stay at his house when I needed a break from living in the car for a day or so.

I lifted, sprinted, conditioned, hit full contact with college players, and trained with Stefon Adams all year. My senior season was going to be *my year*. When it was time for "Hell Week" that year, I was more than ready to destroy everyone in front of me. By the end of my senior year, I'd won every award you could get, including Blue Chip All American, All State, All Southern Section, All Division, All League, and Most Valuable Player.

This "Special Ed Kid" who everyone laughed at signed a full scholarship with the University of Miami, which had just beat Nebraska in the Cotton Bowl to become the number-one-ranked national champion. Plus, I received scholarships to the number two, three, four, and five football-ranked college universities. I said I was going to do it, and I damn well *did it*.

On the last day of high school, I went to see that special education teacher again. I walked into his room and held up the *Los Angeles Times* I had picked up earlier. I told him to read the headline and what it said beneath out loud to me. He read, "Three Area Players Named Football All-Americans" and then "Hochman (6'4 245), who has committed to Miami." We just stared at each other for a long moment. I told him, "Just because you gave up on your dreams, don't ever tell a kid they can't achieve theirs." Then I walked out.

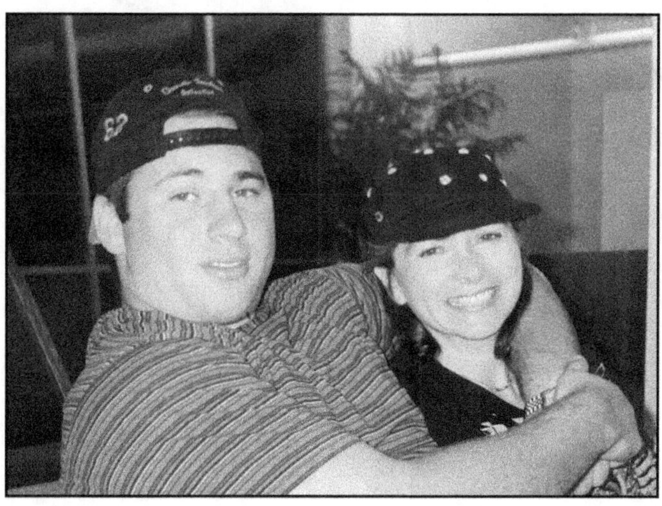

College

I ended up going to college with a lot of guys who went on to become famous, including Warren Sapp, Derrick Lewis, and The Rock, aka Dwayne Johnson.

There I was in Miami, living that freshman life, but it was also the first time I'd lived on my own without my father managing every aspect of my daily routine. I'd achieved my goal of getting a scholarship, but now that I had it, I lacked *purpose*.

Then, two things happened that threw me off course. First, I blew out my ACL during a preseason practice. I still remember hearing a loud "pop" in my knee, then hitting the ground. I had to have knee surgery. Then, as I was recovering from that, my dad told me that he was being accused of check fraud—fraud that he was 100 percent guilty of, not that I knew it since he was conning me too—and if he didn't get $17,000, he was going to prison.

There I was, recovering from surgery, struggling through midterms to keep my scholarship, trying to figure out how to be an "adult," and now I needed to come up with $17,000 to save my father.

I started talking to everyone from the coaches to the boosters (wealthy donors) to try to find this money to save my dad. Meanwhile, I took a bunch of caffeine pills to help me stay awake for an all-nighter while cramming for midterms. The next morning, during a football meeting, I started to feel like my heart was beating out of my chest. My chest was so tight, I could hardly breathe, and they rushed me to the hospital. After running tests and discovering I'd taken the caffeine pills, they said I was having a panic attack.

It was like something broke in my brain. After that, I had panic attacks up to 20 times a day for no reason. It didn't take long for my coaches to realize I wasn't going to make it in Miami, so they suggested I transfer my scholarship to another school.

I ended up transferring to Idaho State University, and they had me playing defensive tackle instead of offensive guard. By then my knee was better, and I had two more years to play football. I was determined to beat out everyone in front of me and become the starting defensive tackle, and I did. Yet whenever we would travel on planes or buses for games, the anxiety became so intense that for hours, I could only take shallow breaths.

The summer between my junior and senior years, I got a job as a bouncer at a strip club. I started dating a stripper, and when the time came for me to go back to school, she came back with me. We ended up getting married, but the relationship was toxic and amped up my anxiety so much that I ended up quitting school and moving in with my wife's grandparents in San Bernadino, California.

There I was, this big white guy living with a Mexican family. When I say I was big, what I really mean is: I was fat. I weighed nearly 300 pounds, and I was filled with anxiety and still without my *purpose* in life. Eventually, my wife and I broke up, and I ended up staying with my father in someone else's tiny one-bedroom apartment in Fontana, sleeping on the floor next to the sofa.

I felt like I was already as low as I could go, and I remember the *exact moment* when I hit rock bottom. I was lying on the dirty floor with nothing but one of those thin, cheap industrial carpets between me and the cement. My dad was sleeping on the couch next to me, and he'd fallen asleep with a lit cigarette in his hand that was about to drop three inches of ash onto my face. The whole place was filthy; I didn't even want to look in the kitchen. I heard gunshots and sirens outside, then I felt something move on my chest. I looked down and saw a huge cockroach crawling on top of me.

I sat straight up, screaming on the inside, "I'm not supposed to be here! I'm not supposed to be here!" That moment changed everything.

The next morning, I called my grandma in Mission Viejo and begged her to let me stay with her. She told me that I could, but there were rules: I couldn't sleep past 6 a.m., I had to be very clean, I had to be home at night by 10 p.m., and I had to have a full-time job. I agreed to everything and dedicated myself to trying to figure out my life.

Fat Albert Got Shredded

I linked up with my friend Albert again, who had graduated and become a microbiologist and chemist, but what was even more impressive to me was that he now had a six-pack! When I last saw him, Albert had been almost as big as I was, but now he was lean, defined, and healthy. I *needed* to know how he did it because I was barely in my 20s but already had extremely high blood pressure. It was high enough that at the rate I was going, I'd be lucky to make it to 50.

Albert taught me about the glycemic index and how insulin works. He explained that if I just ate things that were low on the glycemic index, the fat would melt away. I did what he said, and started a crazy workout regime too—lifting, mountain biking, running, swimming, and mixed martial arts. I didn't *have* to go so hard to get great results—the nutrition changes made my fat melt away—but the exercise was good for my anxiety. Between all that and what I learned from Albert, my body completely transformed.

People at the local 24-Hour Fitness started to notice how fast I was getting shredded. I went from 300 pounds to "Damn, how'd you do that?" in three months. One guy named Paul offered me $100 just to work out alongside me for a week. At the time, I was moving furniture for a consignment store and delivering pizzas, so of course I took the money and let him work out with me. I taught him everything I knew, and he got crazy results too. More people noticed, and the next thing I knew I had a hundred personal training clients.

In just one year I went from being homeless to making $200,000 a year showing people what worked for me to transform my life. I could *never* have predicted or planned this.

BUILDING THE BUSINESS

Within two years, I had a seven-figure personal trainer studio, and I became known as "the six-figure trainer maker."

Trainers all over Orange County, California, came to me to learn my methods. I would teach them, and they would pay rent to train their clients at my gym. My first gym, Next Level Fitness, quickly became the biggest personal training gym in Orange County, with more than 40 trainers.

I ended up opening some of the first indoor fitness boot camps back in 2007, and the concept exploded. A fitness business influencer named Bedros Keuilian heard about me and wanted to create a boot camp business model that could be turned into a worldwide franchise. We partnered up, and I named it Fit Body Boot Camp. We grew it into the biggest boot camp franchise with more than 300 locations in five countries.

On the outside, I looked very successful, but behind the scenes, my personal life was spinning out of control. I was accomplishing my "goals," but I still didn't know my *purpose*. I was also in an unhappy marriage.

It wasn't my now-ex-wife's fault; we just weren't a good match for each other. We met before I discovered the secret to finding your perfect person. You have to *know yourself*—what you require, and what you can give. Without knowing that, it's nearly impossible to match up with the right person.

STARTING FROM SCRATCH, AGAIN

Slowly, I started losing my whole identity, and everything I worked for began to unravel. I had already sold Next Level Fitness and all my personally owned fitness boot camps, so when I got some bad business advice from someone I trusted and sold my half of Fit Body Boot Camp for way under what it was worth, I felt like I had hit bottom again.

After my marriage ended, I decided to open another fitness boot camp in Irvine, also in Orange County, that I named OC|FIT. I simply focused on becoming the person I wanted to be and running my gym.

When something really changes your life, the first thing you want to do is share it with as *many people as possible.* I went from being homeless to figuring out a way to make a living helping people get lean and healthy. I know how much that affected me in a positive way, and I want other people to experience the happiness I have from that.

When you're doing what you love and you're passionate about, it's not work. When I'm really in the zone, helping someone with things that I never used to have but now do, two hours can go by, and I don't even realize it.

A lot of parents will tell their kids to be more disciplined with their lives. They'll tell them to get off their TikTok, which they're "addicted to," and study because it's good for them, because they need a good education so they can move up to the next level and have more opportunities in life. That's great, except that *same parent* will complain about the weight they need to lose—in chronic pain, embarrassed, and unhealthy from it—and then, after making that statement to their kid, walk to the cupboard and grab a cookie because it's right there.

That's hypocrisy. That parent's words won't have the same impact because they don't have the discipline that they're trying to instill in their own kids. You can't give what you don't have. Parenting isn't just about giving value to others, it's living the value that you're giving.

Helping people in as many ways as possible is my purpose, which means I have to be the *best version* of myself in all those ways. You can't give what you don't have. You have to live the value you give if you really want to *bring value* to other people's lives. Once I solidified my purpose, everything fell into place. I ended up meeting Stefanie, my soulmate. She's my perfect match, my everything. As I write this book, we've been together for nine years. In fact, I proposed to and married Stefanie inside the original OC|FIT in Irvine. To be honest, before I found my purpose and did all that work on myself, I wouldn't have been ready for someone of her intelligence, beauty, and caliber.

I continued running and opening up OC|FITs, coaching people on fitness, nutrition, and personal development worldwide, and three years ago, Stefanie and I had our son R.J. Now, I have two daughters (aged 16 and 18 at this writing) from my previous marriage, and R.J. They're all great kids.

The reason I'm sharing my story with you is that I want you to know that you can overcome whatever challenges you might be facing. I was an outcast with Tourette syndrome, a broken family, a con-artist father, paralyzed by anxiety, obesely overweight, had dangerously high blood pressure, and I had been homeless multiple times. All these challenges were hard to go through—even painful—but they were all necessary to allow me to give the most value possible to the people in my life. They made me a better coach, a better father, and a better husband. Now I'm an incredibly healthy, lean, successful businessman with a beautiful and happy family.

I created this life for myself based on the principles I'm sharing with you in this book. You don't need to spend a decade doing more than 10,000 hours to hone and test this system. I did that for you and have made things super easy for you to follow.

The 3 is simple and will cut through all the deceptive food industry's BS and expose the hidden ingredients that are causing you to store fat. You will literally be shocked when you learn what foods and ingredients, many of them considered "health foods," are doing to your body.

This book should be a quick read. It's 100 percent designed for you to get into the right mindset to take *immediate and massive action* on the new knowledge you'll receive. Read it with a positive attitude, knowing that everything you need, everything you've been missing to be the lean, healthy, and unstoppable person you were meant to be, is here for you in this book.

Let's gooooo!

1

Mindset

This chapter is all about sharing powerful mindset habits I've discovered over the years. These are the ones that have changed my life. I was homeless, broke, and obese, but it's not just exercise or nutrition that put me on a successful path. I had to change the way I thought before everything around me started to change.

You might be tempted to skip ahead to the nutrition or exercise sections, but I'm telling you right now: don't. *Mindset* is the *most important* thing you'll learn about in this book. Why is that?

Well, do you currently eat things that you know you shouldn't and regret it afterward? Even after you get the powerful nutrition knowledge I've included in this book, you're still you. You're still the same person who orders dessert and then regrets it on the way home. You'll still mess up and revert back to your old patterns if you don't move beyond simply knowing. A change in mindset is what will give you the ability to implement the new knowledge that you acquire here. I'm going to show you how to *reprogram* your mind so you don't do what I call "breaking character."

This next part might sound strange, but you need to understand that you shouldn't get lean, fit, and healthy just for yourself. If focusing on the benefits to you are your only reasons for making a change, I'm here to tell you that it most likely *will not work*. The reason it won't is because it's too easy and normal to let yourself down. Think about how many times you didn't keep your word to yourself. You didn't show up for yourself.

People abuse themselves all the time without it ever feeling like it's a big deal. Most likely, you would never treat a loved one the way you regularly treat yourself.

Consider a father who constantly lies to his kids. He promises to show up for something that's important to them, and then he doesn't. Week after week, year after year, he continues to *let them down*. Even worse, he says things like, "On Monday, I'm going to start being a good dad and keep all the promises I made," but then on Monday, he breaks his word and lets his kids down *again*. Would you describe this man as a good dad, or a bad person?

This is how most people treat themselves. They let themselves down repeatedly and just deal with it because, well, you're stuck with yourself, and it's happened so much that it feels "normal." But when you don't keep your word to yourself, you lose self-confidence. Without self-confidence, you never even start to believe that you can achieve the thing you set out to do. If you already know you're not going to stick with the exercise program or the new diet, why even bother starting it? And if you can't keep your word about not eating any more fast food, how are you going to have the confidence to do something major, like start a new business or get into a new relationship?

Linking Your Purpose

*"Kids only listen to 10 percent of what you say
and emulate 90 percent of what you do."*

The way for you to succeed at truly changing your mindset is for you to link being fit, lean, and healthy to something *bigger* and *more important* than yourself. If you try to do it just for you, then you're constantly fighting yourself. For instance, maybe you want to get up in the morning and work out every day, but some days you'd prefer to sleep in. You want to be healthy and quit your vices, but you also want to go out and drink with your friends. You want to eat well and be lean, but you also want to grab fast food on the way home.

You want a lot of different things, and if you're just making this change for yourself, then sometimes eating clean and being healthy wins, and sometimes the fast food wins. But when you remove yourself from the equation and make what you do about a *higher purpose*, then the higher purpose wins and you're not the problem anymore.

For me, it's easiest to relate it to being a parent. When you're a parent, you're a leader, and the best leaders *lead by example.* As I like to say, "Kids only listen to 10 percent of what you say and emulate 90 percent of what you do." How can you tell your kids to get off social media, be more disciplined, and start studying if you're also saying you want to get lean and healthy, then reach for that doughnut? It doesn't work.

Any pain in your life that you haven't resolved is being passed on to your kids. You can't give your kids what you don't have. If you don't want your kid to experience what's giving you pain, then you need to solve it for yourself so you can share the solution with them. How do you solve it?

Before you eat that doughnut, I want you to say *out loud*: "For the next few minutes, I'm going to *purposely* hurt my kids." I want you to picture them watching you, seeing you break your word to yourself about what's important to you, while you tell them to be responsible and do what's important for them. Can you do it? I'd be surprised if you could.

Let's say you wake up early in the morning. It's still dark out, and you're up because you're going to get in a workout. You look out your window and see that it's cold, rainy, just awful outside, and you're thinking to yourself, "I'll just work out tomorrow."

Now let's say it's the same scenario, cold and rainy, but you have to pick your kid up from school. There's no way you wouldn't go pick up your kid. And you would never use words like, "I need to get motivated" or "I'll start picking up my kid in school next week, Monday, or the first of the year." It's not even a discussion. Once you relate being fit, lean, and healthy to a higher purpose and see the *direct connection*, doing the right things will be automatic, just like picking up your kid on a rainy day would be.

Once you make the connection to something *greater* than yourself, that's when you'll really start to become a person who can *succeed*. This concept applies to everyone, not just parents. So, really spend some time finding your higher purpose. It might take a while to come to you but because you're now aware, you're on the right track. Until you figure it out, you can adapt my purpose of giving the *most value* to the *most people* in the *most ways*. Wouldn't the world be a better place if everyone had that purpose?

Just remember, you *cannot* give what you *do not* have. So, you have to become the best version of yourself in all the ways you want to give value, especially to your family, friends, and loved ones.

Choose Your Pain, or Your Pain Will Choose You

"Happiness can only exist with contrast."

More people than ever are seeking comfort, and yet more people than ever are depressed. What so many fail to realize is that happiness requires *contrast*—it's the relief from pain, not the absence of it.

Everything in nature adapts to its environment, and *all stimulus* loses its effect over time if it's *constant*. For example, say you work from home. You sleep in late, wake up, then stay in your PJs all day. Instead of working a full day, 70 percent is spent on the couch watching Netflix, sleeping, or eating crap. After "work," instead of exercising, you lay on the couch, binging another series. All throughout the day, instead of eating healthy, you keep your finger on the "pleasure button" by Door Dashing fast food or raiding your cabinet for snacks. You're not even hungry, you just keep eating because you're "bored."

Does this sound like a life of leisure and pleasure? Without contrast, all pleasure loses its effect on your "happiness" and, as you continue to seek constant comfort without contrast, you start to feel *depressed*. The longer you do it, the more depressed you feel. The more depressed you feel, the less you want to do the things that will get you out of your depression.

Finally, you go to the doctor, and they tell you that you have a "chemical imbalance" and give you a prescription to "fix" the problem. But your life is *lacking contrast*, and you're so out of alignment with *who* you really are that no pill can fix you.

For me, I work out partly for the *physical* effect, but the major reason is the *mental* effect it has on me. It makes me feel good—it gives me my contrast. I often start my day with a 33-degree cold plunge. It sucks. I *dread* it. But when I'm done, I feel *amazing*, I'm *proud*, and life seems a lot easier in *contrast*.

Later in the day, I do a hard high-intensity interval training (HIIT) workout. Everything burns, and I'm out of breath, but when I'm done, the contrast feels incredible for hours!

Then, before I go to bed, my wife and I sit in the 200-degree sauna for 20 minutes. By the end, the last few minutes are almost unbearable. But when we get out, collapse on our lounge chairs, and feel that cool air as we lay on our backs looking up at the stars, the contrast has us at happiness level 10.

Now, I'm not saying you have to be as extreme as me. I just don't want you to make the same mistake that I used to make, and millions of others are still making: that seeking perpetual comfort will lead to happiness. I want you to be aware that happiness can only exist with *contrast*. You choose your pain, or your pain chooses you. So, I learned to choose *positive pain* through health and fitness.

You Must Detach to Be Present

*"Detaching gives you a whole new
perspective on everything."*

Being detached does *not* mean that you're not being present in the moment. It's the *opposite*. You're fully present, pretending that you're looking down on yourself from above, fully viewing everything that's happening and how you're reacting and inter-acting. This allows you to detach and watch what's happening so that your response can be less *emotional* and more *strategic*—more aligned with your *conscience*.

There's something about watching an event happening from outside that feels different, like when you watch a movie and yell at the screen for the character not to do something that seems obviously dumb to you. Think about if you had a craving for some candy and you walked over to the cabinet, opened it, grabbed a bag of candy, opened it, reached in, then shoved a handful into your mouth. Doing this would feel way different if you detached and watched yourself have a candy craving, walk over to the cabinet, and do the same thing. You wouldn't be thinking of eating the candy, you'd be yelling at the screen to the main character who was about to *break their word* to themselves. You'd be shouting at the screen, "Noooo, don't do it!"

Detaching gives you a whole new perspective on everything. You must detach to be fully present. It's a *game-changer.*

THINK OF YOUR LIFE AS A MOVIE

"When situations go bad, I say good."

Would you want to see a movie where everything just works out? In the beginning of the movie, everything is good; then, in the middle, everything is good; and when it ends, it's all good.

Would you pay money to see that? I think of my life as if I'm watching a movie and I'm the main character—the reluctant hero. When situations go bad, I say *good*—my movie just got interesting.

Remember what I said about being detached as much as possible—not viewing things from your eyes, but as if you were watching what's happening from above. Little mindset shifts like that can change your whole world, and this little shift in how I look at a situation has changed mine.

So, think of your life as a movie, and make it a *blockbuster*!

If It's Worth Doing, It's Worth Doing Right Now

"If your words aren't congruent to your
actions, the brain ain't buying it."

Everybody says, "I'll start on a Monday." Nobody ever says, "On Wednesday, I'm going to change my life." Let me tell you, nothing kills dreams faster than Monday because Monday turns into the first of the month, and then the next thing you know it's the new year, and on and on. So if anything is worth doing, it's worth doing right now, right here, today. This is one of the reasons why New Year's resolutions rarely work.

I'll show you why you should *never wait* to do something *important.* Let's say your teen came to you and said, "Oh my God! I just realized how much you do for me. You show me so much love and patience. You always support and stand by me, and you make so many sacrifices for me. Yet, I am so disrespectful toward you. I talk back. I don't even do the little things around the house you ask of me. Basically, I haven't appreciated you.

"But that's all going to change. Exactly *one month* from now, I'm going to give you the respect you deserve. Until then, I'll keep acting like a jerk. Or better yet, I'll be a *bigger* jerk, just to get it out of my system before I start being respectful in a month."

If your kid said this to you, you'd know they're full of it because if they were really serious about what they said, they'd *start now.* The subconscious part of your brain works the same way. If your words aren't congruent to your actions, the brain ain't buying it. Besides, if you *really* realized that you're letting *everyone* you love down by not giving them the best version of yourself, you'd change immediately. If it's worth doing, it's worth doing *now*.

> **PRO TIP:** The best time to plant a tree is 20 years ago, but the second-best time is right now. Stop waiting for the perfect time because it will never come. Days of procrastinating turn into weeks, weeks into months, and months into years. Don't seek perfection, *seek action*! Remember, as you walk, the path illuminates.

You don't have to do this alone. Coaching with me is available on my website at www.stevehochman.com.

LIVE A LIFE OF SERVICE

"I had some 'goals' but not a purpose."

For a long time, in so many areas of my life I would fly high, then crash and burn. I'd take two steps forward, then two or three steps back. Finally, one day I figured out the formula not only to stop taking steps back but also to allow me to live a much happier and fulfilled life. The answer was living a life of service.

Most people think that serving others means sacrificing yourself, but it's actually the opposite. I can only give the *solution* to the things that I've *solved*. I can't give that which I don't have. So, I had to elevate myself in the areas that I want to serve. For me, I want to give value in as many ways as possible. If I want to help people with nutrition and mindset, I have to be an *expert* in nutrition and mindset. If I want to help parents, I have to possess and execute high-level parenting skills. If I want to help people with relationships, I have to be in a healthy and loving relationship.

As long as I measure everything I do by asking "can this help me serve others?" I will *always* show up as the best version of myself. People need to receive value, and I have to be of value to give it. It's a beautiful circle! How could I ever let myself get overweight and out of shape when one of the main things I do is help people get lean and fit?

The truth is that most people wouldn't have an answer if you put them on the spot and asked what their *purpose in life* is. How crazy is it that 99 percent of people go through their whole life without ever locking down their purpose? I used to be one of those people. I had some "goals" but not a purpose. It's got to be a worthy purpose, a purpose bigger than yourself. It's very easy to get caught up in having your current feelings or mood dictate your actions, but this isn't the case when you live with purpose, *especially* if your purpose is to deliver value to others.

Here's a crazy story about one of my clients who already understood the value of a life of service but wasn't able to truly live up to his full capacity until he took full responsibility for his health and fitness.

Mike is a 56-year-old hairdresser who owned a hair salon. He started using drugs, and he became so addicted, he began dealing to maintain his habit. As a father and a husband, he grappled with intense guilt for *failing his family* in this way, but he was completely consumed by his addiction.

One night, when he was at home with his daughter, he was the victim of a home invasion. He was targeted because someone had found out that he had cash in his safe from the drugs he sold. Mike and his daughter were held at gunpoint as their hands were zip-tied. However, while the thieves where busy trying to unbolt the safe from the floor, Mike was able to break his zip ties and grab an unloaded shotgun that was behind the door.

Mike racked the shotgun and aimed the barrel at the intruders while screaming for them to get out. Luckily, they ran, not knowing the shotgun was empty. This was the last straw for Mike's wife, and she left him.

Mike's guilt over the traumatic near-death experience he put his daughter through was *unbearable*, and he overdosed on drugs. He was touch and go in the ICU and even had to be resuscitated a couple of times. In his own words:

I had my ups and downs with alcohol and drugs, and in late April 2016, I ended up in the ICU at Saint Joseph's Medical Center in Orange. I had MRSA [Methicillin-resistant Staphylococcus aureus], and my organs were shutting down. After ten difficult days in the hospital, food became an escape for me. I went from 194 pounds to 265 pounds over a period of five years.

I was diagnosed with Stage Four chronic kidney disease, prediabetes, sleep apnea, and asthma. It left me standing in front of the mirror, clean and sober—which I'd worked hard for, as the manager of a sober living facility—but unhappy with how I looked and felt. I called Steve.

Through my personal development program, I pointed out to Mike that he had just traded his addiction to drugs for an addiction to food. I also said that until he became leveled up in all ways, the people he hoped to help at the sober-living facility he runs would never really listen to him because of the unhealthy way he treated his body with food and the physical results of that.

I remember when I was talking to him the first time, and I said, "Wow, great. You got off drugs. Awesome. You cut out a really negative thing. But what positive thing do you have about you that would make someone else want to imitate you? You have a huge gut. Your kidneys are failing. Your liver is shit. You have low self-esteem. Why should anyone listen to you?" He realized I was right and committed to *totally changing* his life.

His motivation for making a change was to live whatever years of life he had left to the fullest. His *higher purpose* was to inspire his daughter and the residents of the sober living house to have a better life through health and fitness and to gain the confidence, pride, and energy that comes along with a life of *self-mastery*.

Together we dove into my program, including mindset work, the 3 Rules, the three accelerators, and workouts. I told him if he sent me his daily food logs without missing a single day, showed up for the weekly calls, and hit the workouts consistently, then everything would fall into place. Mike accepted the challenge, and four months later, he was 50 pounds lighter and completely shredded—you could even see veins on his abs!

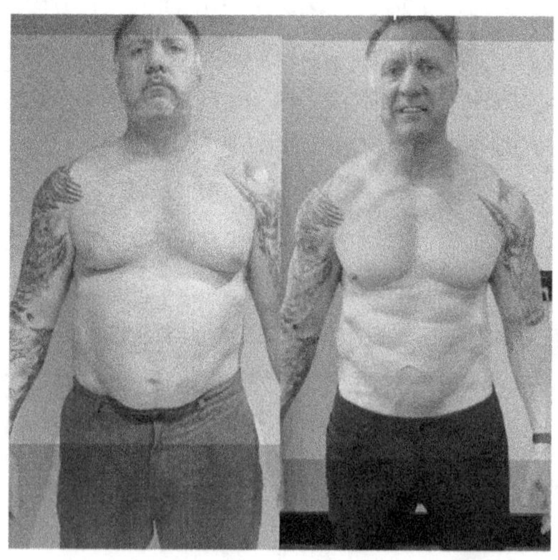

Mike didn't restrict a *single calorie* (no one on my program does). All he did was follow The 3 Rules and work out consistently. I'm so proud of Mike. Not only did he completely transform mentally and physically but his kidneys, liver, and blood pressure are all in the normal range now, and he is no longer prediabetic. Plus, because of the hundreds of people who witnessed Mike's profound and fast transformation, he's been able to help the residents at his sober living house to deeply transform their lives as well. He even got engaged to his dream girl!

Mike's mindset shift allowed him to put The 3 into *action*, which changed his life.

No matter where you're at in life, it's never too late to completely change your trajectory. What's keeping you from starting today? Reach out to me at www.stevehochman.com if you're ready to be your best self!

CHANGE YOUR DEFINITION OF HAPPINESS

"Be aware of the final feeling you
have about anything you do."

Some people say, "When I eat cake, it makes me happy, so I like doing it because it feels good." When you've finished eating the cake, are you still happy, or do you feel regret? What about when you wake up the next morning? Are you still happy about eating all that cake the day before?

We need to change our definition of something feeling good, or making us happy, to how we feel *after*, not during. Whatever the final feeling is, that's what we should label it as.

Even though I work out nearly every day, there are plenty of times I don't want to. There are days I'd love to just binge Netflix instead, and in the moment, it would feel *good*. But afterward, when I reflect on my day, would I still feel good about skipping my workout to lie on the couch?

If I don't still feel good about it, then it didn't make me happy because the final outcome wasn't happiness. Most of your *personal development* comes from simply being *aware*, so be aware of the final feeling you have about anything you do and call it what it is.

Choose Proud Over Happy

*"Only do what makes you proud, and
eliminate what causes you regret."*

It took me decades of struggle to learn this part. We commonly seek two feelings that seem similar but have *very different* outcomes. There's "happiness," which feels good in the moment but requires a karmic debt of pain to be paid later, and "pride," which requires the debt to be paid as you go. Let me explain.

For example, you set a goal the night before to wake up early and workout. Your alarm goes off at 5 a.m. and you decide that it will make you happier to hit the snooze and sleep for another hour. An hour later, you wake up and owe a debt in the form of guilt for not working out, diminishing your confidence because you've yet again broken your word to yourself.

Or the alarm goes off at 5 a.m. and you *choose proud*. You turn the alarm off and sit up. You get dressed and head to your workout. The karmic debt was paid by the pain of overcoming the mental challenge of getting up when you were tempted to sleep.

After the workout, and for the rest of the day, you can feel proud and debt free. If all you get out of this whole book is to only do what makes you proud and eliminate what causes you regret, the trajectory of your life will completely change.

When I discovered this, I started making my decision based on proud. If *this* would make me happy, but *that* would make me proud, I choose *that*.

LET YOUR CONSCIENCE LEAD YOU

"The more you're aware of what your conscience is saying, the stronger that voice gets."

Your conscience is the voice or feeling inside you that's always telling you what to do. It is *always* right and leading you to the path that most aligns with the real you.

Sometimes, we don't follow our conscience because there's so much noise and distraction in our lives that we can barely hear it. Sometimes, we choose to tune it out. But the "voice" of your conscience is always there, and just like the muscles you strengthen from working out, the more you're aware of what your conscience is saying, the stronger that voice gets. *Really* follow your conscience, and every action you take will be the one that's best for you.

Imagine that you know a parent who, every single time their kid gets upset about anything at all, gives the kid a cookie to make them feel better. What would you think of that parent? Would you think they were doing the best thing for their child? Would you think they were making sure their kid grew up happy and healthy?

No, you'd probably think they were a lazy parent for trying to fix every problem their kid ever had with sugar. You'd know that it wasn't a good solution for that kid.

Now take a second to think about yourself. There are easy things you can do to make yourself happy and "solve" your problems, but if you're being honest with yourself, how many of those solutions are just giving yourself a cookie instead of going with what your conscience is telling you? The easiest solution isn't always the right one. Listen to your *conscience* to help figure out what you *should* be doing for yourself, then do it.

BEING HAPPY IS A DECISION

*"Happiness is created by stringing
moments of gratitude together."*

The highest-frequency state you can be in is the state of appreciation or gratitude. Happiness isn't a "destination" that you'll arrive at one day. Happiness is created by stringing moments of gratitude together. How many times a day can I be *aware* of being grateful?

Sometimes, it's hard to feel appreciation for the moment you're in. One powerful method for getting into the state of appreciation is *perspective*. Perspective is when you compare what you're experiencing to someone experiencing something so much worse.

To give me perspective, I think of my teammate Marcus, who was paralyzed from the neck down right in front of me. We were playing college football, and he got knocked out during a tackle. I'll never forget when he woke up. We were all crowded around him, and he had a tear rolling down his face because he couldn't feel anything from the neck down. He had damaged his spinal cord and became a paraplegic for the rest of his life. In that moment, he knew his entire life would never be the same.

When I'm having a bad day, or I'm feeling ungrateful, or things aren't happening fast enough, or I'm mad about something, I think of Marcus. I imagine explaining to him why I'm having such a "bad" day, knowing that he would give anything to have my worst day. My worst day is his *best* day. When I use this perspective, my paradigm shifts, and I'm instantly able to put myself in the state of appreciation for my life.

You may have had experiences or seen things that are way worse than that. *Good.* Use those for perspective. If not, then you can just search YouTube for horrific situations, and use those for perspective. Try it right now. Use perspective. Remember or visualize a *horrific* situation that happened to you or someone else. Now, really *believe* that it's happening to you right now. Make it as real as possible. Hold on to that horrible feeling for 30 seconds. Feel it 100 percent, as intense as you can make it.

As soon as you hit 30 seconds, *immediately* zap yourself back into your life. Pay attention to how many things you are grateful for and hold on to that feeling as long as you can. Constantly find new reasons to feel gratitude. The better you get at this, the happier you will be.

THE GRATITUDE HACK

"Turn on appreciation, and you turn off want."

I believe the universe, or God, or whatever you call it, is like a parent, and we are the children. Think of what I'm going to tell you now from the lens of a parent looking at their child.

It's normal to "want" things. But the more we focus on what we *want*, the more we don't appreciate what we *have*. This is because to think intensely about what we want, we must think intensely about what we lack. It's like an on/off switch. You can't simultaneously want something more and be grateful for what you have. You turn on what you want, and you turn off appreciation. You turn on appreciation, and you turn off want.

Back to the universe being like a parent example ... Let's say you have a five-year-old child who has a whole room of awesome toys, but they come to you and say, "I can't be happy until you buy me brand-new toys." We know that if we get them the new toys, it will only be a matter of time before they come to us again with the same request.

Most parents would try to help their child be *grateful* for the toys they have, and once they saw them doing that, they'd be way more open to buying new toys. I believe this is how the universe works. The universe doesn't give us what we want until we're grateful for what we have (and we've put in the work, too). This doesn't mean we should never want anything. Just like when you want to drive somewhere, you put the address into the GPS and periodically look at it, but you don't stare at your GPS the whole trip, or you'd crash.

So, first you figure out what you want. Next, you make a plan to get it. Then you focus on the work and being in a state of appreciation. Periodically think about what you want to make sure your actions are aligned, but the majority of your time and focus should be on taking action and being in the state of appreciation.

The crazy thing about it all is, the more we think this way, the faster we actually get what we want. Then, when we finally get it, it's just a cool bonus because we didn't even need it to be happy since we're already in such a high *state of appreciation*. Now, we can enjoy what we get without *needing* it to be happy because we already are.

I truly believe that this is the secret to life. When you are in the state of appreciation, you vibrate at a *higher frequency*. People can feel it. The universe can feel it. And you will see it by what you attract the more time you spend in that state.

LIFE IS A MIRROR, NOT A WINDOW (DEALING WITH HATERS)

"Most people aren't ready to change."

A lot of times, when you start making dramatic changes, the people who are closest to you will actually be the ones who try the hardest to pull you down. It's crazy, but I see it all the time. The reason they do this is because life is a mirror, not a window. When someone sees you accomplish something, it's like holding up a mirror where they see their own reflection, and what they may see is a person who's given up or failed at going after their own goals.

So many people have given up on themselves in some part of their life, that when they see you doing what they gave up on, they have two choices. The first choice is to say, "Wow, I'm inspired, I want to do it too. *Let's go!*" Or they could say, "I don't want to put the work in, I'm not ready. So, if I can just make *you* stop, then I don't have to see it, and I don't have to feel bad about giving up on myself." The sad part is a lot of times the negativity comes from the people who are closest to you.

Most people aren't ready to change. They might be afraid, they might be lazy, they might not know where to start—who knows? All you have to do is keep going and know that the only way to deal with haters is with *love*. Rather than feeling attacked, getting angry, or trying to force them to do what you're doing, just send out what you want to receive, which is love. Lead by example.

This is what I mean by giving the most value to the most people. When your transformation becomes *undeniable*, you'll end up helping and inspiring people you didn't even know were watching you!

REGRET AS A MOTIVATOR

"It's never about the what, always about who."

Regret is my biggest motivator and also my biggest fear. I am so scared of getting to the end of my life and having regrets. I don't want to regret any *dream* I had that I didn't pursue. I don't want to regret being lazy when more *discipline* was what I needed. I don't want to regret not doing something because I was uncomfortable or scared. I don't want to wonder what would have happened if I had *given 100 percent.*

You can connect this way of thinking to being lean, fit, and healthy. Let's take identical twins. One is strong from working out consistently, is lean because of the food he eats, and is confident because of the person he's become through the process. The other is physically weak because of choosing to lay on the couch every day and watch Netflix instead of working out, is fat from eating fast food, and doesn't love who he sees in the mirror. Each twin would have a very different trajectory in life. If I were the lazy twin with no discipline, I would definitely regret never fighting for what could have been.

Most people don't give their all because they're afraid of failure. I'm not afraid of failure because I define success as being fully aligned with my conscience. If I do everything I'm required to do for that day, then that day is a win. If I do everything I'm supposed to do for seven days, then I win the week. If I keep going, I win the year, and if I never stop, *I win at life.*

All I have to do to win is three things: follow what my conscience tells me to do, do what makes me proud, and eliminate what I regret. I don't validate myself with anything else. Not the money I have, not the things I have, not what I look like. It's never about *what*, always about *who*.

THE FREQUENCY OF "I GET TO" VERSUS "I HAVE TO"

"Being out of alignment with your conscience,
thinking negative thoughts, or being
ungrateful lowers your frequency."

Everything in nature has a frequency. We've all walked into a room and felt "good" or "bad" energy. The more you are aligned with your conscience, the higher the frequency you vibrate at. Positive thoughts and being in a state of appreciation raise your frequency. Being out of alignment with your conscience, thinking negative thoughts, or being ungrateful lowers your frequency.

One of the mindset techniques I use that quickly allows me to vibrate at a higher frequency is to change the word "have" to the word "get." So, for example, instead of saying, "I *have* to work out" say, "I *get* to work out."

As you say those words out loud, you can feel your frequency *rising*. Saying "I get to" will help you vibrate on a higher frequency because it puts you into a state of appreciation by default. It's a gratitude hack—especially when you're just beginning—to help you raise your frequency and have a more positive mental attitude about the things you're required to do to align with your conscience.

There's No Self-Mastery without 100 Percent Honesty

*"Being honest with yourself is like a muscle
that you develop and strengthen."*

You can never *change* something that you're *lying* to yourself about. If you're making excuses or lying, you have no chance of changing.

Being honest with yourself is like a muscle that you develop and strengthen. At first, it's very difficult and painful to be honest with yourself because you don't want to look at your shortcomings. It's challenging to acknowledge how you're letting yourself down; you don't even want to look at it. But by practicing 100 *percent honesty*, you get good at it, and eventually, lying to yourself becomes harder than being honest with yourself.

Anyone Can Be the Hardest Worker on the Field

*"You can't control how much experience
you have or your God-given talent, but
everyone has an* equal *opportunity each day
to be the* hardest worker *on the field."*

Some people fail to even start working out or eating clean because they think they're too far behind, or just less capable than everyone else. Remember, I started playing football late in the game. I was behind when it came to experience.

A coach once said something that stuck with me. He said, "You can't control how much experience you have or your

God-given talent. But everyone has an *equal* opportunity each day to be the hardest worker on the field. And eventually, the most consistent hardest worker will surpass the person with more talent and experience."

I took what he said to heart and became the best player at my position in the country in just three years. So just focus on you. If you are not the hardest worker, that's 100 percent your choice.

GET UNCOMFORTABLE WITH BEING COMFORTABLE

"People actually love to be
uncomfortable when it's on their terms."

There's nothing that holds people back more than the fear of being uncomfortable. But because I know that no progress is made in my "comfort zone" and the only way I can make progress is by forcing myself to do things that make me uncomfortable, I learned to become *uncomfortable* with being *comfortable*.

To accomplish this, I had to reframe the way I thought about doing things that are uncomfortable. For example, think about going to an amusement park. We get on a roller-coaster, and it scares us to death. It actually mimics the experience of having a panic attack. The difference is, you're *asking* for it. You paid money and stood in line for hours just to get uncomfortable. That's why amusement parks are so packed because people actually love to be uncomfortable *when it's on their terms*.

Over time, I trained myself to seek discomfort. Eventually, very uncomfortable situations that are necessary for progress feel exciting and fun, like being on a roller-coaster!

Being uncomfortable rarely happens to me unintentionally, and when it does, I've programmed myself to *love it*. I seek it out knowing that the more positively uncomfortable I get, the more progress I make. Imagine if for a whole year, instead of avoiding the things that make you uncomfortable, you actively seek them out. How far would you be in just one year?

Now, picture that over a *lifetime*.

I DON'T BREAK CHARACTER

"It's the who, not the what, that's important."

Steve, do you have cheat meals or fall off your 3 Rules? *I don't break character.*

Steve, do you miss workouts? *I don't break character.*

Steve, do you drink alcohol? *I don't break character.*

What about birthdays or family events? *I don't break character!*

The phrase "I don't break character" is such a powerful tool to keep you aligned with your conscience. Your character is linked to who you are and what your purpose is. For example, for me, it's not about being lean. Being lean is just a by-product of my character. Even if who you are now is far from who you *really are* according to your conscience, you can use your character to bridge the gap.

When I see a room full of people at a restaurant who don't like their own naked reflection in the mirror, who want to be lean and healthy, who have promised themselves they will "do better" all while stuffing their faces with junk that they'll regret on the drive home, I see a room full of people breaking character.

When people functioning at a lower frequency try to get me to eat food that will bring me down to their level, and I say "no, thank you," and they keep asking, I love saying, "I don't break character." It's part of a technique called "subconscious auto-suggestion," which I'll go into more detail about later in the chapter.

I don't eat things that are bad for me because I don't want to "break character." Breaking character is an acting phrase that I've adopted and use with my clients. For an actor, breaking character means doing something that the character they're portraying wouldn't do. For example, if you're playing Mother Theresa, we wouldn't see you in a scene abusing puppies.

Because I'm clear about the type of person I want to be, I don't break character by eating food that doesn't align with my conscience. I help the people I work with do the same thing. Here's what my client Alex has to say:

Growing up in Colombia, soccer was a big part of my life, and staying physically fit came naturally. However, over the years, I became comfortable in my marriage and lifestyle, and my weight gradually increased to nearly 300 pounds. I found myself eating without ever feeling truly satisfied, and I relied on multiple energy drinks a day just to keep up with my routine. I knew I needed to make a change.

After some research, I discovered Steve and OC|FIT. From the moment I connected with Steve, I sensed that this coaching program was something special. I was eager to learn as much as possible because the 3 Rules just made sense. For the first time, I no longer felt like I was on a restrictive diet. I stopped weighing my food and counting calories, and instead focused on eating until I was satisfied and fueling my body with healthy, unprocessed foods that support fat loss. The system is truly set up for success.

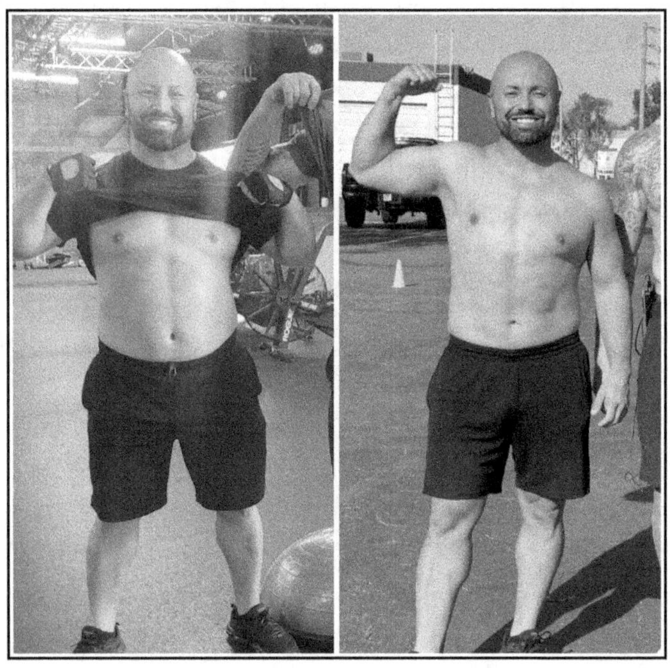

I've had clients tell me "I went to a concert, but I didn't drink any alcohol because I didn't want to break character." When I start to hear them say things like that, then I know they've *finally* got it. It means they understand it's not the food or the drink they're focusing on—instead, it's who they want to be that they're working toward. It's the who, not the what, that's important.

OVERCOME YOUR ANXIETIES

*"The gap between where you are and where
you know you could be is where anxiety lives."*

In the introduction, I shared how I overcame crippling anxiety. There are a few things I learned from that time that I apply to my life now. First of all, I realized that a lot of times anxiety is just *excess energy* that needs to escape the body. I found that doing HIIT workouts really helps me to burn off that extra energy.

Another thing that helped me was simply working harder in all aspects of my life. I realized that if I could work myself hard in business, in parenting, in my relationships, in mentoring, and of course in working out, then I would burn off all that energy. Yes, I'm pretty exhausted at the end of the day, but I'm *proud*.

Finally, I realized I'd never be fully free of anxiety if I wasn't aligned with what my conscience was telling me to do. If your conscience is telling you to be something better than what you're doing, you will *always* be in a state of anxiety. It might be low level, or it might be high level—whatever it is, you'll never be at peace if you're not aligned with your conscience.

You might be saying, "I'm a good parent, I'm a good person, I make a lot of money." Great, but if you're overweight and it's bothering you, then you know you could be better. The gap between where you are and where you know you could be is where anxiety lives. Closing that gap means becoming better at being the real you—your *best self*.

One of the benefits of being your best self, totally aligned with your conscience, and proud of who you are, is that when you walk into a room, your energy and your presence are just different because you've done the work. You're challenging your weaknesses every day and you're proud of yourself in all aspects of your life. You should be. Believe it or not, that's rare.

Looks Matter

"If you don't look right, it's because something isn't right."

You're not getting fit just to look a certain way; getting fit is part of the process of becoming the best you. However, *looks do matter* because the outside is a representation of the inside. You wouldn't even be reading this book if I was 50 pounds heavier. You're reading this book because I'm super fit. I'm 50 years old with a six pack, but I used to weigh 300 pounds. I know what it feels like to be on the other side of the coin when it comes to your looks.

If you don't look right, it's because something isn't right. Something about you doesn't add up. It's like if you're looking for someone to help you manage your finances. You find two people with the same credentials and good track records and schedule meetings with them. If one financial manager shows up in a filthy, broken-down car with duct tape on the windows while the other pulls up in a Rolls Royce, who are you going to choose to work with? The one who *looks* like a success!

When a person walks in a room, they give off an *energy*. We've all felt it when we walked into a place and said, "Oh, this place has bad energy" or "I like that person; they have good energy." Many people don't give off their full potential of energy because they are out of alignment with their conscience. Your conscience is the voice or feeling you get inside when you are doing something that is not aligned with the *best version* of yourself. When you go to dinner and stuff down that dessert, the guilt you feel is coming from your conscience letting you know you are out of alignment. Basically, when you just don't feel good about yourself, you'll give off that low frequency energy that people can feel.

The Importance of Confidence

*"Confidence is earned through keeping your word
to yourself and maintaining your daily habits."*

I've already mentioned confidence in a few different places so far, but it's important enough to really focus on here. We know that a confident person is infinitely more successful in all ways than someone who's not confident. Confidence is something you have to earn. When you can't even do the little things, you're not confident that you'll be able to do the big things. It's not even about the "physical" appearance, it's about the *thought process* that led to what you see on the outside.

There is no question that an overweight person has an area of their life, one they care about, in which they're completely undisciplined. *That* is what's unattractive—seeing a person who can't seem to stop doing something that they are not proud of and is making them unhealthy. We know it, they know it, and their *energy* is congruent to it. You show me someone who's put in the work, created daily habits, and is proud of themselves in all ways, and I'll show you someone who is emitting loads of confident, high-frequency energy that people are attracted to.

On the other hand, when you can't keep your word to yourself, even for the little things, you can't truly be confident—especially for the big things. Let's say you want to start a big business, but you can't even get to the gym on time. You can't even get up early, like you said you would, to work out without hitting that snooze button. You say you'll stop eating junk, but you stop for fast food on the way home. If a friend lied to you as much as you lie to yourself, you'd want nothing to do with them because you wouldn't trust them. You would *not* have confidence in them.

That's why you lack that powerful, confident mindset. Because you've lied to yourself so many times. Raising the frequency of your energy and your confidence starts with keeping your word to yourself until you've built self-trust, and thus self-worth. Many people go their whole lives without ever realizing this important fact. Confidence is earned by keeping your word to yourself and maintaining your daily habits.

That's one huge reason why eating right and keeping up with your workouts is important—this is you proving to yourself that you can follow through. That's why the people who become successful in one area tend to succeed in other areas. If you want to increase your confidence, do the little things your conscience is telling you to do. This will give you an inner confidence and determination that will amp up your powers of manifestation.

THE POWER OF SUBCONSCIOUS AUTO-SUGGESTION

*"Subconsciously, your brain will suggest
those words when you need them."*

Remember me mentioning subconscious auto-suggestion a few pages ago? It's one of the things that really helps me in my life. Subconscious auto-suggestion is saying certain words repeatedly in certain circumstances to the point that, subconsciously, your brain auto-suggests those words when you need to hear them in the right situation.

For example, if you associate eating the correct foods to your character, and every time you go to eat the wrong foods, you say to yourself, "I'm not going to break character, I'm not going to break character, I'm not going to break character." Then, eventually, when you go to some event, like a wedding, and they bring out the cake, your brain tells you, "No, I'm not breaking character. I'm not breaking character."

FOLLOWING THE 3 IS JUST THE BEGINNING

"Always anchor your goals to a higher purpose."

I know we've spent a lot of time on mindset, but the truth is that winning over your weaknesses or falling prey to them is all decided in your mind. I want you to win in all areas of your life, that's why I've written this book. To me, developing the right mindset is the foundation for victory, and it will make it easier for you to follow The 3.

However, the rules work with or without a perfect mindset because it's just science. Here's a story about another client whose transformation I supported that proves this point.

I've long struggled with my weight, finding it difficult to maintain a healthy range regardless of whether I was underweight or overweight. When I got really heavy, I would resort to starving myself to lose weight. However, I always ultimately gained back even more, with my highest weight reaching 265 pounds. At that point, I was prediabetic and dealing with chronic kidney issues.

I explored various options, including weight loss pills, injections, and restrictive eating, and even received a referral for surgery from my endocrinologist. This was the moment that it became clear to me I needed to make a change; I was exhausted from feeling unwell both mentally and physically. I didn't recognize myself in the mirror and regretted allowing my health to decline to that level. I was frequently ill, often requiring hospital visits, and even simple tasks like climbing the stairs in my apartment left me breathless. I knew it was time to seek answers and take control of my health—not just for me, but so I could be the active, engaged mother my kids deserved.

When I met Steve and learned about his 3 Rules, I was intrigued from the very start. It was a turning point for me when I realized that this approach was something I could share with my entire family. My kids embraced the 3 Rules, and they genuinely enjoy the meals I prepare! I'm pleased to share that I've successfully addressed the kidney issues I once faced and am no longer prediabetic. I feel healthier than ever and continue to grow stronger each day. I'm more present and engaged in my roles as a wife, mother, and friend, and have become a better version of myself.

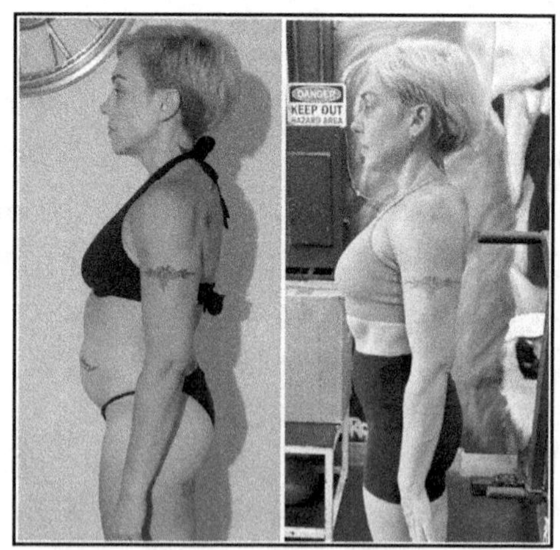

One of the most powerful shifts for Laura was that we stopped focusing on the *what* and started focusing on the *who*. Who is Laura? Laura is an example for her kids, she's the ultimate wife for her husband, and she's proud of who she is today.

Never be held back or defined by the limiting beliefs of the people around you. Surround yourself with a tribe of positive, motivated, and knowledgeable people who bring out the best in you. Don't *ever* diminish your worth.

To recap:

- A strong mindset is *essential* to create real, lasting change.
- You need to connect your goals to a *higher purpose* than just yourself.
- Become the *best version* of yourself to provide real value to people you care for. It's never about the *what*, always about the *who*.
- Continuous comfort makes you *bored* and *depressed*; you need contrast to really appreciate what you have. Deliberately making yourself uncomfortable is how you grow.
- Don't think about exercise as something you *have* to do. Think about it as something you *get* to do.
- Real change is impossible unless you're *honest* with yourself.
- *Anyone* can be the hardest worker on the field. Hard work overcomes natural talent any day of the week.
- Your conscience is the voice or feeling inside you that's always telling you what to do. Really follow your conscience, and every action you take will be the right one.
- Real confidence comes from keeping your promises to yourself. Failing to follow through on those promises breaks down your trust in yourself.

- Surround yourself with people who help bring out the best in you, not tear you down.

In the next chapter, you're going to learn Rule 1 of The 3—Stay Below 25 on the glycemic index. The glycemic index is the most powerful tool for nutrition you've never heard about. Get ready to stop weighing your food, counting your calories, and starving yourself. Staying below 25 on the glycemic index is the most important thing when it comes to your nutrition, and I'll explain how to do that without denying yourself delicious and flavorful foods.

2
Rule 1—Stay Below 25 on the Glycemic Index

If you do nothing else in this book but follow Rule 1 for the rest of your life, you will be *leaner* and *healthier* than most people—all without having to weigh your food or count calories. Rule 1 says to stay below 25 on the glycemic index (GI). For that to make sense, though, you need to understand the GI.

WHAT IS THE GLYCEMIC INDEX ANYWAY?

Rule 1 is the primary rule of the whole program. I wish there were another, less scientific name for the glycemic index—you could call it the sugar scale or something—but we're just going to call it the GI.

The GI is a measurement that relates to how quickly what you consume causes your blood sugar (glucose) to rise. The higher the number, the faster your blood sugar goes up. For example, table sugar has a glycemic index of 65, so your blood sugar rises super-fast, while broccoli has a GI of 10, so it goes up very slowly.

When your blood sugar rises quickly, your body releases insulin to remove glucose from your bloodstream and store it in your cells. When your blood sugar rises slowly, like when you consume foods and ingredients below 25 on the GI, you get a much lower insulin release.

Insulin Is Your Most Powerful Fat Storage Hormone

When insulin is present in your bloodstream after eating, it makes you absorb glucose—sugar—and other nutrients in your cells. Think of insulin like a key that unlocks the door to your cells so glucose can be stored inside of them.

Why is this important? This is actually the key to Rule 1—your cells use glucose for energy, and insulin is the hormone that moves that glucose into your cells. Extra glucose is stored in your liver, muscles, and *fat* cells. However, when you eat foods below 25 on the GI, there's so little insulin released that it *virtually eliminates* fat storage.

Most people don't bother to manage their insulin levels unless they're diabetic. If you're not managing your insulin levels and you're trying to lose weight, you likely think the best option is to lower your calories. I was talking to a client recently, someone who's pretty fit but still not quite there. She wanted to know how to get leaner. I told her about the 3 Rules, and she said, "Oh, I've worked with a nutritionist before, so I kind of know how to eat. I've done macros." But the problem, she said, was that when she got leaner, she always lost her curves. She didn't want to get rid of her booty, so she'd change the way she ate to get her curves back and gain some muscle, but then she had too much body fat again.

So, the problem was that when she was in a big enough calorie deficit to get lean, she would lose muscle along with body fat. That calorie deficit was unsustainable and didn't even give her the body she wanted. I knew that if she were to just cut off the fat storage mechanisms, she could eat enough food to maintain and even build muscle while losing body fat and keeping her curves. To do that, she needed to understand the magic number of 25 on the GI.

I said, "Okay, so when you stop getting leaner and you want to keep going, what does your nutritionist do? What adjustments do they make?" And she said, "They lower my calories."

"That's right. So they lower your calories, then you lose more body fat, right?" And she said, "Yes."

"What else do you lose?" She said, "Muscle."

"Then when you get stuck again, what do they do?"

"They lower my calories."

I said, "Okay, so what's happening here is you're doing something that's working on one aspect of your nutrition, but *not* working on two aspects. So, the aspect that's working is that you're losing fat when you cut calories, so that's great, but you're also losing muscle—that is, your curves—and you're slowing down your metabolism and setting yourself up for future failure because your body is now continually adapting to being in a very low, restrictive calorie deficit. Your body doesn't know that you're in a city and not in the jungle, so it's constantly adapting to the lower calories by slowing those metabolism mechanisms down, *slowing down* the fat-burning process because it thinks you're going to need that.

"And what happens is eventually, when you're so sick of starving yourself just to lose fat, only to be upset because now you lost your curves, when you go back up, your metabolism is even slower than it was before. Now, when you do eat enough food to gain the muscle and the curves back, you're getting even more fat than you had before, and you're *stuck* in the cycle of cutting and bulking, cutting and bulking and never, ever being fully satisfied with your body or able to sustain this year-round."

WHY IS IT SO IMPORTANT TO STAY BELOW 25 ON THE GI?

I was always close, but after two decades, I finally nailed down the *magic glycemic number* of 25. Foods with a GI under 25 have a minimal impact on your blood sugar levels. This means your body doesn't need to release a flood of insulin—the hormone responsible for fat storage. When blood sugar stays stable and insulin remains low, your body is free to burn fat for energy instead of locking it away in your fat cells.

In simple terms, keeping your GI low creates the perfect environment for fat loss.

When you eat foods over 25 on the GI, you get glucose and insulin spikes, and this means *fat storage*. When your blood sugar rises quickly (as it does with high-GI foods), excess glucose is stored as fat. This is your body's way of saving energy for later—except that later almost never comes.

By focusing on foods under 25 GI, you avoid these *fat-storing spikes*. As a result, shockingly less fat is stored, and more of what you eat is used as energy to fuel your body. This means your body becomes a *fat-burning machine*, making it easier to stay lean and have energy.

Staying below 25 on the GI is like flipping a switch in your metabolism—it stops storing and starts burning.

One of the most surprising things my coaching clients discover when they start following The 3 is that they usually **under-eat**—not because they're trying to but because they're just **not as hungry**.

High glycemic foods spike your blood sugar and send it crashing back down. That crash is what triggers those intense hunger signals, even when your body doesn't really need more food.

By sticking to foods under 25 on the GI, blood sugar levels stay stable all day long. No spikes. No crashes. No cravings. This stability naturally reduces your appetite.

When you eat foods higher than 25 on the GI, you trigger the reward centers in your brain, making you crave even more high glycemic food. It's a horrible cycle.

The right GI fuel makes all the difference. When you're eating following The 3, your body burns fat efficiently and sustains energy for longer. It's like upgrading your metabolism to premium fuel. You're no longer eating to "refuel" every few hours—you're powered up and ready to go.

OBVIOUS HIGH GI FOODS AND INGREDIENTS

The "scientific" definition of low on the GI is anything under 55, medium is 56 to 69, and high is anything above that. That would make table sugar, which has a GI of 65, medium on the GI. Does that mean if you just chowed down on a bag of sugar, you could consider that part of a medium GI diet? Could there be a diet worse than that? That makes *no sense* to me.

Say you're one of the few people in the world that actually kind of understands that the most powerful tool for getting lean is the GI, and you venture out on the internet to try to learn about it, then see values like that. It might make you feel justified to eat anything 55 and under on the GI because that would be considered low! You'd eat that way, then wonder why you weren't getting lean.

If you're wondering how the "experts" could have gotten it so wrong (and if you research the health ministers for most countries, you probably won't see really fit people), just look at the food pyramid. According to the food pyramid, the majority of what you're eating would be ultra-processed foods with the very ingredients that are causing obesity and feeding metabolic diseases. If you asked almost anyone, "Hey, if your diet is mostly bread, cereal, rice, and pasta, do you think you'll be lean or fat?" Ninety-nine percent of people out there would probably say, "Well, you're definitely not going to be lean."

It's the same with the GI. The GI is just a scale between 0 and 100, with 100 representing glucose. But the scientists who gave everything else numbers weren't thinking about what was going to make you lean. They saw the halfway point on the scale and decided that would be a good cutoff point for "low" on the GI, but this is an insignificant number when it comes to your health.

If you're reading this book, you're looking to *lose fat* and *be healthy* without having to do all the things that you failed at before, like counting calories, calculating macros, or starving, while having fun and *loving* what you eat. That's what I'm here to help you do, and that's why I'm telling you the number you need to get results.

Look, I'm someone with subpar genetics when it comes to gaining weight—I'm not blessed to be lean no matter what I eat. I was really fat before I figured The 3 out, and now I'm shredded at age 50, and have been for the past *24 years*, personally training *thousands* of people along the way. I have tested the number 25 on the GI for more than two and a half decades, and I know it works.

Obvious Foods

There are lots of foods that people know aren't good to eat if you want to lose body fat. (Don't think you can never eat these, though—I'll show you how to have them all the time The 3-Rule way.) Some that are commonly known are the following:

1. **White bread**—GI ~75–85
2. Sugar (table sugar)—GI ~65
3. High fructose corn syrup—GI ~87–100
4. **Donuts**—GI ~75–95
5. Pastries (croissants, danishes)—GI ~70–80
6. **Cake**—GI ~70–85
7. **Cookies**—GI ~70–80
8. Ice cream (sugary varieties)—GI ~60–80
9. **Soda/soft drinks**—GI ~60–75
10. **French fries**—GI ~70–95
11. **Sugary cereals**—GI ~70–90
12. **Candy**—GI ~70–100
13. **Energy drinks**—GI ~60–75
14. **Pizza (white dough)**—GI ~60–80
15. **Bagels (white flour)**—GI ~70–90

NOT-SO-OBVIOUS FOODS

These are not-so-obvious because a packaged food can say "zero sugar," but as you can see below, you still get an insulin response, which gives it the same, or worse, fat storage effect. It doesn't matter if it's organic, non-GMO, or some other "healthy" buzzword—you're still not going to get lean eating it.

1. **Honey**—GI ~58
2. **Brown rice syrup**—GI ~98
3. **Coconut sugar**—GI ~54
4. **Dates**—GI ~62
5. **Ripe bananas**—GI ~51

6. Dried fruits (like raisins)—GI ~64
7. **Quinoa**—GI ~53
8. **Pasta (white)**—GI ~45–50
9. **Whole wheat bread**—GI ~69
10. **Whole wheat pasta**—GI ~48–58 (depending on the brand and preparation)
11. **Potatoes (baked)**—GI ~85
12. **Instant oatmeal**—GI ~79
13. **Sweetened yogurt**—GI ~36–50 (depending on sugar content)
14. **Couscous**—GI ~65
15. **Barley**—GI ~66
16. **Rice cakes**—GI ~82
17. Pancakes (made with white flour)—GI ~66
18. **Muffins** (store-bought)—GI ~57–68
19. **Granola bars**—GI ~50–70 (depending on ingredients)
20. **Cornflakes**—GI ~80–90
21. **Popcorn (plain)**—GI ~65–85
22. **White rice**—GI ~70–90
23. **Puffed rice**—GI ~80–90
24. **White crackers**—GI ~70–80
25. **Pretzels**—GI ~80–85
26. **Fruit snacks**—GI ~70–80
27. **Jams and jellies**—GI ~65–80

THE HIDDEN INGREDIENTS

These ones are way less obvious because most people haven't heard of them, but they're everywhere. So many people are consuming these hidden ingredients daily without even knowing it, feeding their diseases and making them fat. In one of the top brands of stevia, which is an all-natural, 0-glycemic sweetener, the first ingredient isn't even stevia. It's maltodextrin, which has a glycemic index that's *higher* than sugar.

It's just one more sneaky way the food industry can give you less—"zero sugar"—without making you any healthier. They get record profits, and you get *addicted, fat*, and *sick*.

1. **Dextrose**—GI ~100
2. **Maltodextrin**—GI ~105–110
3. **Tapioca starch**—GI ~70–90
4. **Potato starch**—GI ~85–100
5. **Modified food starch** (various types like corn, potato, or rice)—GI ~85–100
6. **Cornstarch**—GI ~85–100
7. **Rice starch**—GI ~95–100
8. **Wheat starch**—GI ~70–85
9. **Arrowroot starch**—GI ~70
10. **Sago starch**—GI ~85
11. Cassava starch (similar to tapioca starch)—GI ~70–90
12. **Amaranth starch**—GI ~97
13. **Sweet potato starch**—GI ~70–90
14. **Barley starch**—GI ~60–65
15. **Sorghum starch**—GI ~70
16. **Pea starch**—GI ~65–70
17. **Glucose syrup**—GI ~100
18. **Corn syrup**—GI ~90–100
19. **Brown rice syrup**—GI ~98
20. **Fruit juice concentrates** (e.g., apple juice concentrate)—GI ~65–70
21. **Polydextrose**—GI ~70

How to Find the Glycemic Index of Everything

Finding the GI of practically any food or ingredient is easy. Just Google "The glycemic Index of (food/ingredient)." Nine times out of ten, the glycemic index will pop up.

ChatGPT is another really good way to find the GI of foods. You can actually just copy and paste a list of ingredients and ask it to list them in the order of high to low on the glycemic index. In the paid version, you can actually take a picture of ingredients and just have it list them out for you. Think of how easy it would be to see if a food was under 25 on the GI that way.

For anyone who's still thinking that this sounds like a lot of work, it won't be a lot of work forever. After a couple weeks, if you really look up the ingredients of everything you eat, honestly, you'll have learned the value of 90 percent of everything you're ever going to eat for the rest of your life.

Let me repeat this: in two weeks you'll know if nearly all the ingredients that you're ever going to need are a *Go* or *No Go*.

You have to look up each food and ingredient—*you* have to do the work, and I already showed you how to do it fast and accurately. You have to arm yourself against the food industry that's trying to make you unhealthy and dependent. Instead of the nutritional facts, if every package of food stated the GI and you stayed below 25, everyone would be lean and 90 percent healthier.

You have two choices. You can do what you're doing now: not be aligned with your conscience, gain weight year after year, and be left with no choice but to practically starve and hope you see some progress. Or you can follow The 3 and make yourself into a *leaner, fitter,* and *healthier* person than you've ever dreamed you could be.

PREVENTING DIABETES WITH THE 3

*"Type 2 diabetes is not only
preventable—it may be reversible."*

More than 37 million Americans have diabetes (about 1 in 10), and approximately 90 to 95 percent of those people have type 2 diabetes, which most often appears in people over age 45, but more and more children, teens, and young adults are also developing it.

In my experience, most cases of type 2 diabetes can be prevented—and in many situations, I've seen it significantly reversed through lifestyle and nutrition changes. You develop diabetes from an overuse of a hormone, which is insulin. Just like anything in life, you adapt to it. That's why you get calluses after doing something for a long time, or if you do the same workout every day, it eventually stops having an effect on you. If you're overusing insulin by giving yourself multiple insulin spikes every day, eventually your body becomes *resistant* to the effects of insulin.

What happens then? Well, your body produces more and more insulin to have less and less of an effect. Finally, your body can't produce enough of it to get your blood sugar to go down, and so you have to start taking medications to reduce your blood sugar, like synthetic insulin. What I've consistently observed is this: When people follow The 3, they dramatically reduce the need for insulin throughout the day. As a result, their sensitivity to insulin improves..

Even in those already diagnosed with diabetes, I've seen remarkable improvements. Some have been able to get off medications entirely, and their doctors are stunned at how well their numbers have normalized.

HOW TO INTERPRET THE GLYCEMIC INDEX

The reason I went from obese to lean so quickly and have stayed that way for 25 years while helping 1,000 people and counting get the same results is because I use the K.I.S.S. method—Keep It Super Simple. That means sticking with the plan. As a rule, if *any* ingredient in the food I want to eat is over 25 on the glycemic index (GI), the food is a No Go if I can't eliminate or replace those ingredients (with the exception of Rule 3, Strategic Carb Timing, which I'll break down later).

For example, if something has five ingredients and four of them are 10 on the GI, and one ingredient is 80, then it's a no go.

PRO TIP: The 3 Rule ice cream compared with a regular, popular brand:

Regular ice cream is made with some ingredients that are over 25 on the GI and cause Glucose > Insulin > Fat storage. These ingredients are:

Milk—~31 (Contains lactose, a natural sugar)

Sugar—~65 (High GI, spikes blood sugar fast)

Skim Milk—~37 (Higher GI than whole milk due to lower fat content)

Versus the 3 Rule ice cream:

Low-Fat Cottage Cheese—~10

Whey Protein Powder—~0–10

Liquid Stevia—0

Unsweetened Almond Milk—0

It's all about the ingredients, *not* the calories. One version makes you store fat, the other does not. The difference between getting lean and gaining fat usually comes down to one or two ingredients that can be easily swapped out.

There's no diet or lifestyle that won't be drastically improved by following Rule 1. Reid is a 28-year-old copywriter who I hired to write an email campaign about The 3 method. He's always been an athlete and even ran track in high school. He consistently works out and watches what he eats. He was in decent shape, but he didn't have a six pack.

I said, "Why don't I just coach you for 30 days, and then you can write about your firsthand experience." He told me that he would do it, but he didn't think there'd be a big difference because he already lifts weights and eats "healthy." I smiled and said, "Just watch."

Reid had an *amazing* transformation. Here's what he has to say about his experience.

Before starting the Three Rules and the Fat Shred program, I honestly didn't know what to expect. With so many nutrition plans out there, I was overwhelmed, but this program felt completely different—so I went for it. From day one, I felt like I was "cheating" because the food was so delicious, yet the fat just kept melting away. And the best part? I was eating more than I ever had on any other plan!

Most programs make you believe you need to cut calories to see results, but here I was, eating more and seeing my body transform. Years later, I'm still lean, still have the six-pack, and people in the gym even ask if I'm on performance enhancing substances, lol! This program was one of the most impactful parts of my fitness journey. Thank you for a life-changing experience!

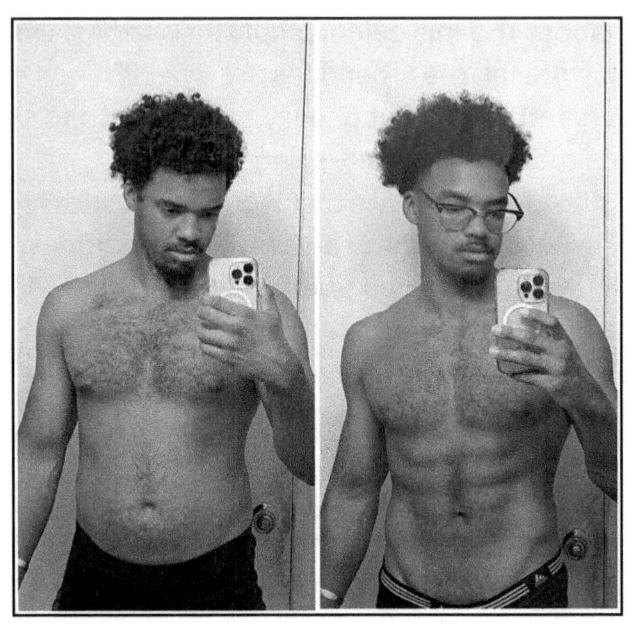

Reid was *never happy* with his body before The 3. He was starving to get lean and losing muscle, decimating his metabolism and feeling hungry 24/7, or bulking (dramatically increasing calories) to gain muscle, but also getting fat. Once he learned and applied Rule 1, Reid was able to eat much more food for muscle gain while, at the same time, seeing his six-pack come in because he wasn't storing fat. This solution and way of life is *so obvious*, yet *no one* is talking about it.

What if you're vegan? Just because you're eating a plant-based diet doesn't mean that the GI doesn't apply to you. I've met many overweight and *unhealthy* vegans, and most vegan alternative meats are nothing but heaping helpings of ultra-processed, fat-storing, addictive, inflammatory ingredients. If you go to the store to buy high-quality beef, there's one ingredient: organic grass-fed beef. But if you buy fake beef, it's got tons of ingredients like starch, dextrose, food dyes, and palm oil. It's not healthy.

The same with Keto. If you choose to follow a Keto diet, you need to know the GI to know if you're *really* doing a Keto diet. If you just rely on the label the food industry puts out there, then you go buy keto bread that has the first ingredient of modified wheat starch? That's high on the glycemic index, which is the complete opposite of being Keto. Not to mention, the moment you get kicked out of ketosis, all the fat you've been eating and using for fuel will end up getting stored in your cells instead.

By the way, none of the terms *Paleo, Keto, net carb*, and the like are regulated at all, leaving the food industry able to lie and deceive you with no consequences.

Don't get fooled by clever marketing of all the different "diets" out there. Just because it bills itself as healthy doesn't mean it actually is. Look at a cauliflower pizza crust. Here's the first four ingredients in the cauliflower crust I found at the store: water, rice flour, tapioca starch, and rice starch. We haven't even *gotten* to cauliflower yet, and everything except the water has a GI over 50.

The 3 Rules cut through all the noise, but you've got to do the research on what you're eating yourself to be sure every ingredient is under 25 on the GI.

However you live your life, whether you just do the 3 Rules and nothing else, or apply the 3 Rules to any diet that you're on, following The 3 is the *best way* to live if you want to be the fittest, strongest, and healthiest version of you.

Here are some common "health" foods that claim to be good for you yet contain ingredients that are way over 25 on the GI.

BOTTLED MINT TEA

Always check the ingredients, even for drinks that are thought of as healthy.

1. Filtered water—GI 0
2. Organic yerba mate—GI unknown, likely low
3. Organic peppermint leaf—GI unknown, likely low
4. Organic spearmint leaf—GI unknown, likely low
5. Organic rooibos leaf—GI unknown, likely low
6. Organic rose hips—GI unknown, likely low
7. **Organic cane sugar—GI 65 (Similar to table sugar or candy)**
8. Organic yerba mate extract—GI unknown, likely low
9. Organic lemon juice concentrate—GI unknown, likely low
10. Citric acid—GI 0
11. Organic caffeine—GI 0

GLUTEN-FREE PRETZELS

A lot of times people confuse gluten free with "healthy." As you can see in these pretzels, you're walking into a glycemic nightmare, with four of the ten ingredients being higher than table sugar. Always check the GI of each ingredient until you get good enough to just know.

1. **Cornstarch—GI 85 (similar to pizza crust or doughnuts)**
2. **Potato starch—GI 90 (similar to pizza crust)**
3. **Tapioca starch—GI 85 (similar to pizza crust or doughnuts)**
4. Palm oil—GI 0

5. Sodium carboxymethylcellulose—GI unknown
6. **Dextrose—GI 100 (similar to Coke or high-fructose corn syrup)**
7. Salt—GI 0
8. Sunflower lecithin—GI 0
9. Baking powder—GI 0
10. Yeast—GI 0
11. Citric acid—GI 0
12. Soda—GI 0

BBQ Sauce (Sugar-Free)

Sometimes it's just one ingredient that really doesn't fit. In this case, it's that sneaky corn starch. Food companies put it in so many things as a thickening agent. Always know each ingredient or look it up.

1. Water—GI 0
2. Distilled vinegar—GI 0
3. Apple cider vinegar—GI 0
4. Allulose—GI 0
5. **Corn starch—GI 85 (similar to pizza crust or doughnuts)**
6. **Tomato paste—GI 38 (similar to ketchup)**
7. Salt—GI 0
8. Fruit juice color—GI unknown
9. Natural flavors—GI unknown
10. Spices—GI unknown
11. Onion powder—GI 0
12. Garlic powder—GI 0
13. Steviol clycosides—GI 0

GRAIN-FREE TACO SHELLS

Don't get fooled by buzzwords. The two primary ingredients in this product are cassava flour and cassava starch. Both ingredients have a higher GI than table sugar. Always check the ingredients yourself.

1. **Cassava flour—GI 72 (similar to chips or white bread)**
2. **Cassava starch—GI 85 (similar to pizza crust or doughnuts)**
3. Avocado oil—GI 0
4. Pumpkin seed meal—GI unknown, likely low
5. Pumpkin powder—GI unknown, likely low
6. Psyllium husk powder—GI unknown, likely low
7. Sea salt—GI 0

PALEO PANCAKE AND WAFFLE MIX

Here's a popular brand that *claims* to be healthy, but the GI exposes that it's actually a blood glucose bomb. Check the glycemic index of all ingredients.

1. **Tapioca starch—GI 85 (similar to pizza crust or doughnuts)**
2. **Organic coconut sugar—GI 54 (similar to table sugar or candy)**
3. **Potato flakes—GI 90 (similar to pizza crust)**
4. **Sweet potato flour—GI 70 (similar to chips)**
5. Leavening (monocalcium phosphate, baking soda)—GI 0
6. Salt—GI 0
7. Guar gum—GI 0

Cookie Dough Keto Bites

It *cannot* be Keto if one of the main ingredients is over 85 on the GI. No matter what it says on the front of the package, always turn it around and check the GI of the ingredients.

1. Organic roasted cashews—GI 15
2. **Organic prebiotic tapioca—GI 85 (similar to pizza crust or doughnuts)**
3. Organic cocoa butter—GI 0
4. **Organic coconut milk powder—GI 45 (similar to whole-grain bread)**
5. Sea salt—GI 0
6. Organic monk fruit—GI 0
7. Organic roasted macadamia nuts—GI 15
8. Organic pea protein—GI 0
9. Pure water—GI 0

Chocolate Chip Cookie Granola

This comes from a company that used clever marketing to brand itself as "healthy." I personally know so many people who eat this with no idea how unhealthy it actually is. They see ingredients like maple syrup and coconut sugar that have been touted as smart sugar alternatives. But the GI doesn't lie. Always check the GI and make sure all ingredients are in line with the 3 Rules regardless of a brand's reputation.

1. **Organic certified gluten-free oats—GI 55 (similar to white bread)**
2. **Organic coconut sugar—GI 54 (similar to table sugar or candy)**

3. **Chocolate chunks (cane sugar)—GI 65 (similar to candy)**
4. **Maple syrup—GI 54 (similar to table sugar or candy)**
5. Chicory root fiber—GI 0
6. Organic chia seeds—GI 1
7. Leavening (cream of tartar, baking soda)—GI 0
8. Sea salt—GI 0

ORGANIC ORIGINAL OAT MILK

Oat milk is quickly becoming a popular "healthy" alternative to cow's milk and almond milk. I hear people saying all the time that they switched to oat milk because it's "healthier." You may be shocked to find out that the GI of oat milk is 70, which is *higher* than pure table sugar. This is because the oats are broken down by enzymes into maltose, which has a GI of 105. Always check the GI!

1. Filtered water—GI 0
2. **Organic gluten-free oats—GI 55 (similar to white bread)**
3. Himalayan pink salt—GI 0

WHEAT KETO BREAD

I checked the ingredients in a very well-known brand of bread billed as being one of the healthiest. The GI doesn't lie, but unfortunately marketing agencies do.

1. Water—GI 0
2. **Modified wheat starch—GI 85 (similar to pizza crust or doughnuts)**
3. Wheat protein isolate—GI 0
4. Sunflower flour—GI unknown, likely low

5. Vegetable oil (soybean)—GI 0
6. Yeast—GI 0
7. **Maltodextrin—GI 100 (similar to Coke or high-fructose corn syrup)**

STEVIA (RAW)

I don't know how they get away with it. You use Stevia to *avoid* the negative glucose spiking effects of sugar. But this popular brand sells Stevia that's cut with dextrose. Dextrose is a highly processed simple sugar with a glycemic index of 100, which is 35 points higher than table sugar. I don't know how this is even legal. Check the GI no matter what.

1. **Dextrose—GI 100 (similar to Coke or high-fructose corn syrup)**
2. Stevia leaf extract—GI 0

ALMOND FLOUR CHOCOLATE CHIP COOKIES

All "made with almond flour" means is that there is some almond flour in the ingredients. It doesn't even mean it's the main ingredient, as you can see in the list below, which is in order of most to least abundant. There is little to no difference between these cookies and regular ones. Always check the GI of the ingredients.

1. **Tapioca starch—GI 85 (similar to pizza crust or doughnuts)**
2. **Chocolate chips (cane sugar, unsweetened chocolate, cocoa butter)—GI 65 (similar to candy)**

3. **Organic coconut sugar—GI 54 (similar to table sugar or candy)**
4. Nut and seed flour blend (almonds, organic coconut, flaxseeds)—GI 1–15 (similar to nuts or seeds)
5. **Arrowroot—GI 67 (similar to white bread)**
6. Vanilla extract—GI unknown
7. Sea salt—GI 0
8. Baking soda—GI 0
9. Cream of tartar—GI 0
10. Rosemary extract (for freshness)—GI unknown

CAULIFLOWER CRUST FROZEN PIZZA

This is another great example of how "made with" doesn't mean "made of." With four out of five of the main ingredients being higher GI than table sugar, you might as well just eat regular pizza. Clever branding might be saying one thing, but the GI will always illuminate the truth.

1. Crust (cauliflower)—GI 15 (similar to nonstarchy vegetables)
2. **Brown rice flour—GI 68 (similar to white bread)**
3. **White rice flour—GI 72 (similar to chips or doughnuts)**
4. **Corn starch—GI 85 (similar to pizza crust or doughnuts)**
5. **Tapioca starch—GI 85 (similar to pizza crust or doughnuts)**
6. Vegetable oil (canola, sunflower, or olive oil)—GI 0
7. Egg—GI unknown, likely low
8. Baking powder (sodium acid pyrophosphate, sodium bicarbonate, corn starch, monocalcium phosphate)—GI 0
9. Xanthan gum—GI 0
10. **Sugar—GI 65 (similar to table sugar or candy)**
11. Yeast—GI 0

12. Vinegar—GI 0
13. Salt—GI 0
14. Sauce (water, tomato paste, seasoning blend [granulated garlic, spices, onion], salt, granulated garlic, basil)—GI unknown
15. Low moisture part-skim mozzarella cheese (pasteurized part-skim milk, cheese cultures, salt, enzymes)—GI unknown, likely low
16. **Tomatoes—GI 38 (similar to ketchup)**
17. Parmesan cheese (pasteurized milk, cheese cultures, salt, enzymes)—GI unknown, likely low
18. Basil—GI 0

MOTIVATION MOVING FORWARD

Remember when you first learned to drive? Getting on the freeway was so scary and confusing. How is this going to work? Should I go faster or slower? You were anxiously checking your mirrors and looking over your shoulder as you hoped for a safe opening in the traffic. In the beginning there were so many things to think about! It was uncomfortable and probably a little scary—especially if you live in a big city.

Fast-forward to now, after you've been driving for a while, getting on the freeway is no big deal. Do you even think about it? If we're being honest, you might even be texting and steering with your knee. The point is, that's how *any* new thing in life is. You don't quite know how to do it; you're nervous and scared, and it's uncomfortable (we talked about that in the Mindset chapter). Then, after a while it becomes second nature. Just follow The 3, and soon you'll find it so easy you could teach it!

To recap:

- Rule 1 is: Stay under 25 on the GI.
- The GI measures how quickly what you consume causes your blood sugar to rise. The higher the number, the faster your blood sugar goes up. The more it rises, the more insulin your body releases, and the more glucose is stored as fat in your cells.
- Staying under 25 on the GI means your body releases so little insulin that very little fat is stored in your cells.
- The technical definition of a "low glycemic index" food is anything under 55. This definition has no science behind it related to *fat storage and metabolic health*—it's just a midpoint on a scale. Decades of testing have proven to me that a truly low GI diet is eating foods under 25.
- There are obvious, not so obvious, and hidden high-glycemic ingredients in the foods we consume on a daily basis. Cut these out by consuming foods and ingredients that are under 25 on the GI .
- Look up the GI of *every food and ingredient* you eat using apps like ChatGPT and Google. After 2 to 3 weeks, you'll know what ingredients are over 25 and will rarely have to look them up.
- Staying under 25 on the GI is one of the best ways to improve your insulin sensitivity, which can lead to preventing or even curing type 2 diabetes and many metabolic diseases.

3
Rule 2—Do Not Combine Carbs and Fats in the Same Meal

I discovered Rule 2 several years ago when I started intermittent fasting. I kept everything I ate the same—the only difference was that I went 16 hours without eating, and then ate all my meals in an 8-hour eating window. Other than that, I changed nothing.

The strange thing was that I started gaining body fat. I couldn't understand what was happening. I went deep into the research and discovered that when you break an extended fast of 16 hours or more, your body produces an insulin spike *no matter what you eat.*

Since I was breaking my fast with scrambled eggs with avocado and cheese—protein and fat—the insulin being released to absorb the glucose out of my bloodstream and into my cells was also absorbing and storing the fat. When I switched to breaking my fast with less than five grams of fat, I *immediately* started seeing results.

I started experimenting with my wife and my coaching clients. I kept all their food the same, apart from not letting them eat carbs and fat together in the same meal. I changed nothing else. Across the board, the results were undeniable.

Redefining Carbohydrates

If you ask 99 out of 100 people "What happens to your body when you eat a lot of carbs?" they're going to say, "It makes you gain a lot of weight." If you go a step further and say, "Why?" they'll probably say, "I don't know. Maybe it's the sugar?"

The reason why carbs make you gain weight is because of their glycemic index (GI). If the food is over 25 on the GI, you release a lot of glucose into your bloodstream, then your body releases insulin to absorb the glucose and stores it as fat. But the problem with this is that we're making a blanket definition of what a carbohydrate is.

Let's take the macro nutrients of cooked broccoli and red potatoes. Because they both have virtually no fat or protein, they are both technically "carbs." But what they do inside your body is very different. This is because broccoli has a glycemic index of 10, while red potatoes are about 90.

Both red potatoes and broccoli will cause some glucose and insulin release—but at *completely different levels*, and with a *completely different* fat storage outcome.

Here's how it works:

Red potato (High GI ~89)

Breaks down *fast* into glucose.

Causes a *big* insulin spike.

Floods the bloodstream with glucose.

Insulin rushes in to pull that glucose into cells.

Glucose gets converted to fat for storage.

Broccoli (Low GI ~10)

Breaks down *very slowly* into glucose.

Barely causes any *insulin release*.

Glucose enters the bloodstream *gradually* and in tiny amounts.

No major insulin response—almost nothing compared with a red potato.

Virtually no fat storage.

So since carbs under 25 GI have a very different effect than carbs above 25 GI, and 99 percent of the time we are talking about "carbs" in relation to gaining or losing weight, I have redefined "carbs." I've never met someone whose problem was they're eating too much broccoli to get lean. So, over the years, I've redefined a carb to mean anything over 25 in the glycemic index, since that's what's going to make you store fat, and anything under 25 GI is just called "food."

There's so much misinformation out there about nutrition. I hear people saying over and over again that they heard you should have fat with carbohydrates to slow how fast your body digests the carbs, which "lowers" the blood sugar spike. The problem with this is that it doesn't slow it down enough. It's like the difference between getting hit by a car at 80 mph versus 60 mph—either way, it's bad!

A lot of times people feel like they have to have carbs and fat together or else, they'll feel hungry. What I discovered is that when you're consistently having insulin spikes throughout the day, your cravings are going up and down all day long. This yo-yo effect intensifies the craving mechanism in your mind.

Another thing I've found that really helps with cravings is being hydrated. The part of your brain that tells you you're hungry is the same part that tells you you're thirsty. It's very difficult to tell the difference between the two signals. A lot of times, we misinterpret being thirsty for being hungry.

Like I said, this isn't meant to be a science book, it's an action book, so if you want to know the science behind Rule 2, I've got you: just go to www.stevehochman.com.

For example, I wouldn't combine steak and rice in the same meal. The GI of standard white rice is 70–89, and although there's a lot of protein in steak, a typical 6-oz top sirloin has 19 grams of fat. I'd swap the white rice out for red lentil rice or air-fried green vegetables. Another example would be combining peanut butter and an apple. Two tablespoons of peanut butter have 16 grams of fat.

Figuring this rule out is the "a-ha" moment for some of my clients. Here's what Shula has to say about it:

When I started Steve's program, I was recovering from a knee injury, so I couldn't do as much physical activity as I wanted, but I still wanted to give it a try. I had tried other diets and exercise programs in the past, but I still wasn't getting the results I wanted.

Once I learned The 3, it was a game-changer for me! It only took me a couple of weeks to learn and understand his rules, specifically Rule 2, not combining carbs and fat. Steve explained that since everyone thinks about "carbs" for losing body fat, he redefined a carb as anything over 25 on the glycemic index. Anything under 25 is just "food." It made sense when he explained it to me like this: table sugar and broccoli are both carbs, but one makes you store fat and the other doesn't, so they're really nothing like each other. He said I didn't need to worry about combining carbs and fat as long as the food was 25 or less on the GI.

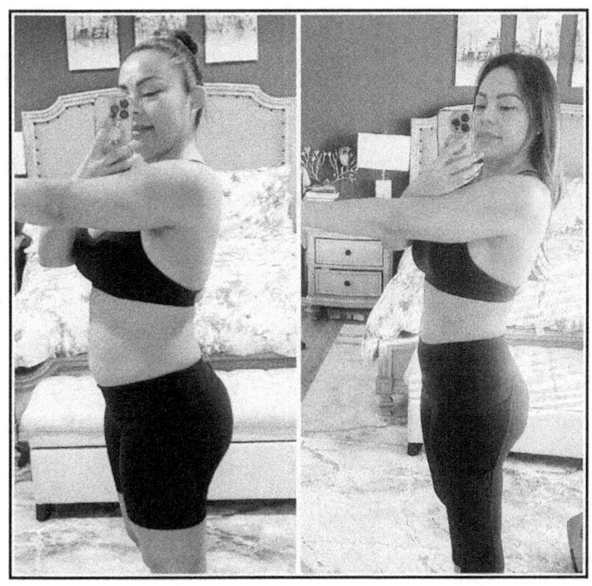

If you're following Rule 1, "Stay under 25 on the glycemic index," then you really don't have to worry about Rule 2. The only time this rule will affect you is in Rule 3, Strategic Carb Timing, which I'll explain in the next chapter. For now, you just need to know that if a food or ingredient is over 25 on the GI, it's considered a carb, so don't have fat with this meal, including one hour before or one hour after because it takes about that long for your insulin levels to drop.

We don't want fat in your bloodstream at the same time an abundant amount of insulin is present. Insulin is the body's primary fat-storage hormone. If you eat something with both fat and carbs at the same time, the glucose in the carbs will trigger insulin being released into your bloodstream, and then your body is going to go into overdrive storing all those nutrients, including fat, in your cells.

Here's another story about one of my coaching clients who was able to completely transform her life and her body just from following The 3.

Amy was a 40-year-old, extremely overweight schoolteacher. She had tried every "diet" out there. In fact, when I met her, she was in one of the most popular weight loss programs in America. Of course it didn't work because this program is just a way to manage your calories, but practically every meal breaks at least one of the three rules and is loaded with ultra-processed ingredients. Maybe you'll lose a little weight, but you're going to consume a lot of ultra-processed, addictive ingredients, and probably never hit your goal anyway because you can only restrict your calories for so long. Amy was no exception, and she was convinced that there was no hope for her.

The first thing I did was connect her fitness goals to her higher purpose. As an elementary school teacher, she really wanted to have the most positive impact on her students as possible. Over the years, she'd seen firsthand how childhood obesity and diabetes had increased exponentially. But, if she was part of the problem, how could she be part of the solution? Amy also had kids of her own, and she was afraid that if she wasn't able to guide them and lead by example, they'd have a higher probability of becoming another negative statistic.

Now that we had her higher purpose anchor, I showed her The 3 Rules and Accelerators and told her to send me a daily food log so I could add another layer of accountability and make sure she was doing everything right.

One of the biggest things that I help with when it comes to the food logs is that when someone breaks character and cheats, I can give them an alternative that falls within the 3 Rules. For example, when I saw that Amy was eating chocolate at night, I asked her about it. She said that when she got stressed, she turned to chocolate, especially late at night when she had a deadline. She said she couldn't imagine giving up chocolate for the rest of her life.

I told her that she didn't have to. I let her know about a sugar-free, low glycemic brand of chocolate chips. I told her, "Now you can get lean while eating delicious chocolate without the guilt or negative effect." I think she was so happy she nearly cried. You'd have thought I had just gifted her a new car.

Over the next six months, Amy lost over 50 pounds and became a role model of health for her students and kids.

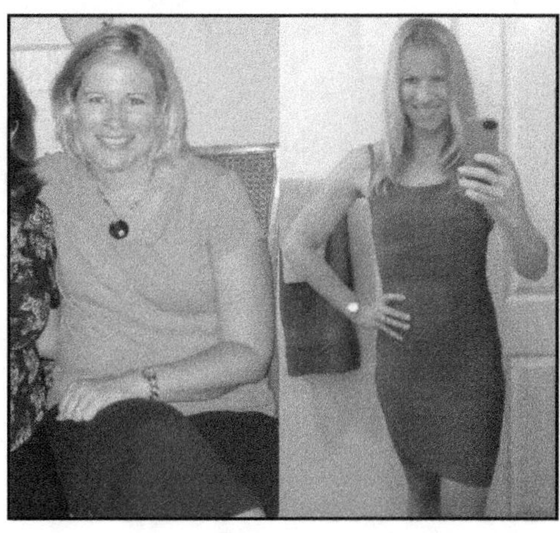

To recap:

- Rule 2 is: Don't combine carbs and fats in the same meal.
- Carbs are defined as foods with a GI over 25. If it's under 25 on the GI, it's just food.
- You can eat foods under 25 on the GI like chicken, broccoli, and steak with fat, but not foods over 25 like fruit, potatoes, and rice.

4

Rule 3—Strategic Carb Timing (aka SCT)

Up until this point, you might be thinking you'll never eat foods like fruit, potatoes, pasta, rice, or bread ever again. Take a breath. There is a specific time, once a day—on the days you work out (so work out often)—when you can and *should* have carbs. (And remember, carbs = any food or ingredient over 25 on the glycemic index.)

This is where **Strategic Carb Timing (SCT)** comes in.

WHY SCT WORKS

Strategic Carb Timing is exactly what it sounds like: timing your carb intake strategically for maximum benefit. That means you should be eating your carbs for the day right after your workout, when your body is primed to replace glycogen (stored glucose in muscle cells) and repair broken-down muscle fibers. This perfect timing for recovery and muscle growth, and the SCT meal tastes *amazing*!

When you work out, you:

- Break down muscle fibers (which need repairing to grow stronger)
- Deplete glycogen stores (which need replenishing for energy recovery)

To rebuild stronger, your body goes through protein synthesis—the process of repairing and growing muscle fibers. But for this to happen *effectively*, your body needs three key components:

1. Two Types of Carbs: Starch and Glucose

Your SCT meal should include two specific types of carbohydrates:

Starch (slow-digesting carb)—Think red potatoes, sweet potatoes, or white rice. These replenish muscle glycogen steadily and provide sustained energy.

Glucose (fast-digesting carb)—Think *blueberries, strawberries, or other fruits*. These quickly restore glycogen and spike insulin to drive nutrients into muscle cells for recovery.

2. Protein (Preferably Whey Protein)

Carbs alone aren't enough. Your muscles need amino acids from protein to rebuild. Whey protein is ideal because it digests quickly, flooding your system with the amino acids necessary for protein synthesis. This *super charges* muscle repair and growth *immediately* after training.

3. (Optional) A Base

To make your SCT meal taste like a *post-workout reward*, you can include a base like fat-free Greek yogurt or a blended shake. This isn't required, but it helps with texture and flavor.

Lori and Cleydi: From Food Struggles to Food Freedom

Lori and Cleydi are both moms and high-level executives. Being Type A can mean having an *all-or-nothing mindset*—especially when it comes to food. When you don't fully understand what to eat, you tend to undereat and avoid foods you don't understand. Food becomes the enemy—so eating less feels like battling fewer enemies. Life becomes about *deprivation* instead of thriving.

Lori's Story:

Before The 3, I'd feel good for a couple of weeks counting calories and tracking macros ... but then, it got exhausting. I'd eventually give up and go back to cereal and fast food. Then came the guilt. To "fix" it, I'd start skipping breakfast and lunch—only eating after 3 p.m., hoping it would make me feel better. But it was NEVER sustainable.

When I started The 3, everything changed instantly. I stopped stressing about portions because I was focused on ingredients instead. I used Steve's recipes, looked up the GI, and FINALLY felt confident in my food choices—free of guilt. I ate the foods I LOVED, just swapped out the bad ingredients for good ones. I could even still have some of the carbs I used to crave with my SCT meal, which helped me feel like I wasn't deprived.

And even though I was eating MORE than ever before, I kept getting leaner and more toned. The other night, I was lying in bed and felt hard bumps on my stomach. I called my husband over, and he looked at me and said ... "Those are

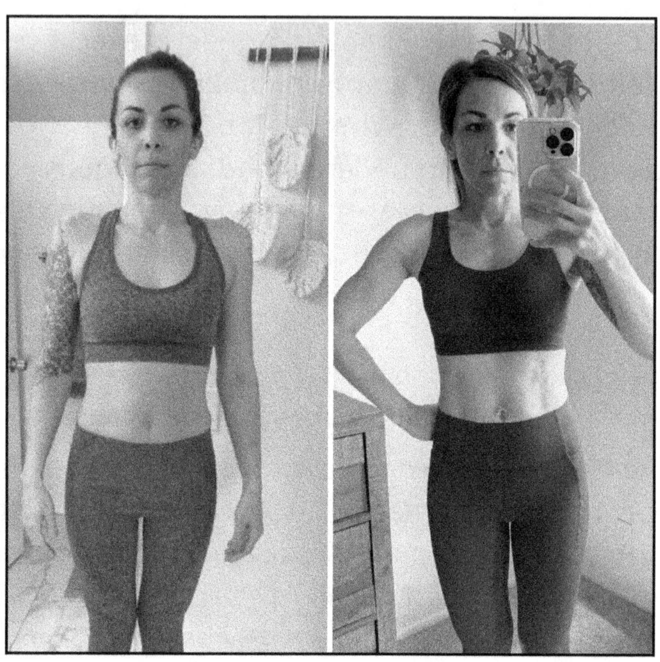

Cleydi's Story:

My relationship with food has always been a stressful one. I tried EVERY diet out there, and never felt happy or satisfied. I thought being lean meant constant restriction. I just accepted that suffering through hunger was the ONLY way.

Then I got on The 3, and Steve asked me to send him a few days of my food logs. He took one look and said, "I know exactly what the issue is." Then he explained the GI and the 3 Rules ... and it made TOTAL sense. I changed the

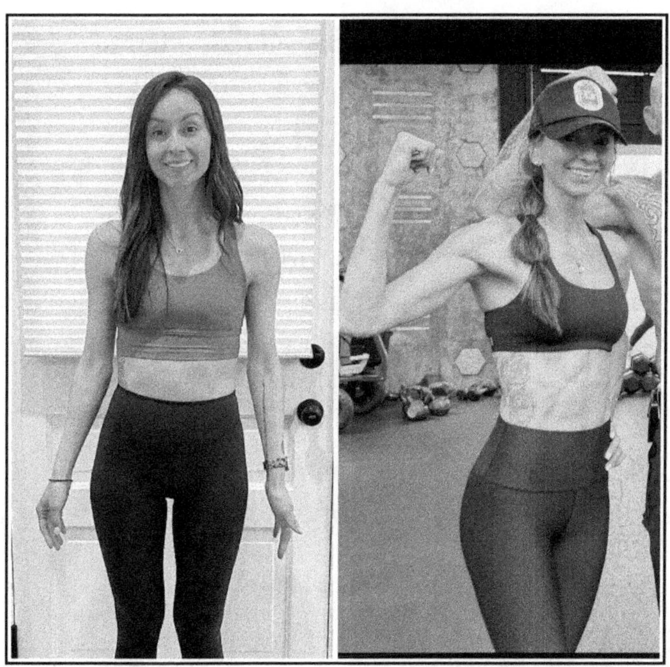

KEEP FAT MINIMAL (UNDER 5 G)

It's crucial to keep fat intake low in your SCT meal—*no more
than 5 g of total fat*. Why? Because this post-workout meal is the
one time per day you will *intentionally* have a glucose and insulin
spike. The insulin will shuttle nutrients (amino acids and protein
for protein synthesis, and glucose to replace the glycogen you
depleted) into your muscle cells.

If fat is present in excess, insulin will store it along with glycogen, leading to unwanted fat gain instead of pure muscle recovery. This is why your SCT meal should focus solely on protein and the right carbs—keeping fat to no more than 5 g.

WHAT HAPPENS IF YOU SKIP SCT?

If you work out and don't replenish glycogen or provide protein for muscle repair, you risk:

- Slower muscle recovery
- Increased muscle soreness
- Weaker performance in future workouts
- Loss of muscle over time
- Not having a "rewarded" feeling after, or a "pumped" feeling during your workout.

Your body is primed to absorb and use these nutrients post-workout. Missing the window means missing out on optimal recovery.

WHAT HAPPENS IF YOU EAT TOO MANY CARBS (ANYTHING OVER 25 ON THE GI) THROUGHOUT THE DAY?

Outside of the SCT window, your body isn't as efficient at using carbs for recovery. Instead, excess carbs throughout the day can lead to:

- Unwanted fat storage (since insulin levels stay elevated longer than needed)
- Blood sugar spikes and crashes

- Increased cravings and energy crashes
- A host of metabolic diseases

This is why SCT is the only time of day you strategically consume carbs.

> **PRO TIP:** Since insulin is the most powerful absorption hormone, the best time to take vitamins and most supplements is with your SCT meal.

HOW MUCH CARB AND PROTEIN SHOULD YOU HAVE?

The general guideline is:

Protein: ~25–50 g whey protein (depending on your size and training intensity)

Starch: ~1/2 to 1 cup cooked red potato, sweet potato, or white rice

Glucose: ~Approx 1/2 cup blueberries, strawberries, or another fruit

You don't need to overcomplicate it—just aim for a balance of these components.

(For more SCT meal ideas, see the "Recipes chapter" or go to www.SteveHochman.com.)

WHY ONLY ON WORKOUT DAYS?

Your muscles only need this carb refill when they've been depleted through training. If you eat SCT-style meals on rest days, you're adding carbs without the demand for them, which increases the risk of fat storage instead of muscle recovery.
    No workout? No SCT meal.

TIMING: HOW SOON AFTER A WORKOUT?

The best time to have your SCT meal is as soon as possible after training, ideally within 30 to 60 minutes. This is when your muscles are most insulin-sensitive, meaning they'll soak up the nutrients quickly and efficiently.

WHAT IF YOU CAN'T HAVE YOUR SCT MEAL RIGHT AWAY?

If you can't eat right away, don't stress. If you eat it within 2 hours, you'll still get most of the benefits. If it's been more than 2 hours, your muscles may not absorb glycogen as efficiently, but the meal will still help recovery. If you expect it to be a long delay, then at the very least, have whey protein immediately after training, then get your carbs in when you can.

WHAT IF I WORK OUT TWICE PER DAY?

Just pick one workout, and have your SCT after it. Whether you work out one time or three times per day, just have one SCT meal.

SCT Meal Examples:

Whey protein + red potato + blueberries (classic, easy option)

Fat-free Greek yogurt + whey + blueberries + diced sweet potato (smooth and creamy texture)

Protein shake with whey, blueberries, and cooked rice (fast and portable)

To recap:

SCT is simple:

- Only eat carbs post-workout.
- Use two types: starch and glucose.
- Pair them with protein.
- Stick to this rule and watch your recovery, strength, and leanness improve.

The **SCT meal** isn't a free pass to binge on carbs—it's a strategic tool to rebuild muscle, restore energy, and optimize performance. Follow it consistently, and you'll see the results.

5
The Accelerators: How to Supercharge Your Results

The accelerators are additions to The 3 that will help you kick your fitness, and particularly your fat shredding, into *high gear*. They're not absolutely necessary if you're following The 3, but using the accelerators will do just that—accelerate your progress. Who wants to get results more slowly? Think of it like buying a sports car. It already goes fast and performs amazingly well, but if you turbocharge it, it'll go even *faster*.

Everyone, no matter where they are in terms of goal and progress, should stay hydrated and curb their cravings with the Magic Fat-Shred drink. It's the best recipe I've found that will do both of those things for you.

The 36-Hour Fast focuses on burning fat, plus it increases your sensitivity to insulin so that your body needs to release less to get the same result, which means less fat storage. It's a great way for people with diabetes or who are prediabetic to cure their illness faster. It's also a good reset if you've had a cheat weekend or didn't do well on a holiday.

And intermittent fasting enhances everything just a little bit, but if I could only choose two, I would choose the first two.

ACCELERATOR #1—THE MAGIC FAT-SHRED DRINK

A lot of times when you feel hungry, you're really thirsty. This is because the same part of your brain that sends signals when you're hungry is also the part that tells us we're thirsty. It's called the hypothalamus.

Over the past 20 years, I've developed the perfect drink for hydration, fat burning, and craving crushing. I call it the Magic Fat-Shred Drink.

One of the most important parts of hydrating is to *want* to drink water. And for that to happen it has to taste amazing. It also has to have a high absorption rate.

The Magic Fat-Shred Drink does more than just hydrate. It helps mobilize fat from your fat cells. It took me many years of research and real-world experimenting with myself and my coaching clients to come up with the perfect formula that tastes amazing, hydrates more, and helps with food cravings.

I conducted experiments on myself where, for a month at a time, I would keep my diet exactly the same, and change just one ingredient of the formula at a time, then take note of what happens. With this final recipe, I noticed I got a little leaner. I was already really lean, so it wasn't a dramatic difference, but it was enough to know that I had the right formula.

I then started experimenting with my coaching clients. First of all, they *loved* the taste. They said that it helped them drink a lot more water because it was so delicious. They also said it helped lessen their intense cravings for food, which made sense because they were more hydrated, and like I said, a lot of times we confuse the signals for thirst with hunger cravings.

Dina was one of my OC|FIT boot camp members. She had been working out for years and was super fit and strong on the inside. However, she just appeared to have a normal "mom bod" on the outside.

The accelerator that helped Dina was the Magic Fat-Shred Drink. Dina had struggled with strong cravings all her life. Since your hypothalamus sends signals for both hunger and thirst, sometimes those signals get crossed. We feel starving, but we're really just thirsty. Being super hydrated can help *crush* those cravings. Because the Magic Fat-Shred Drink tastes so good and hydrates you so well, a lot of times those strong cravings disappear.

When Dina first came to me, she wasn't convinced by it. In Dina's own words:

I'd tried every diet out there—counting calories, low-carb, and everything in between. Either it didn't work, or I couldn't stick to it. So, when Steve introduced his 28-Day Fat-Shred program, I was skeptical. I'd tried so many approaches, and I was starting to think my goals were just out of reach.

But with Steve's coaching, for the first time, I had a nutrition plan I could actually stick with—and the results were amazing! In just 28 days, I lost nearly 20 pounds and got leaner and more defined than I've ever been in my life. Years after I first did Steve's program, I'm still lean and muscular, and checking the glycemic index has become second nature. At 56, I'm in the best shape of my life. Thank you, Steve, for showing me what's possible!

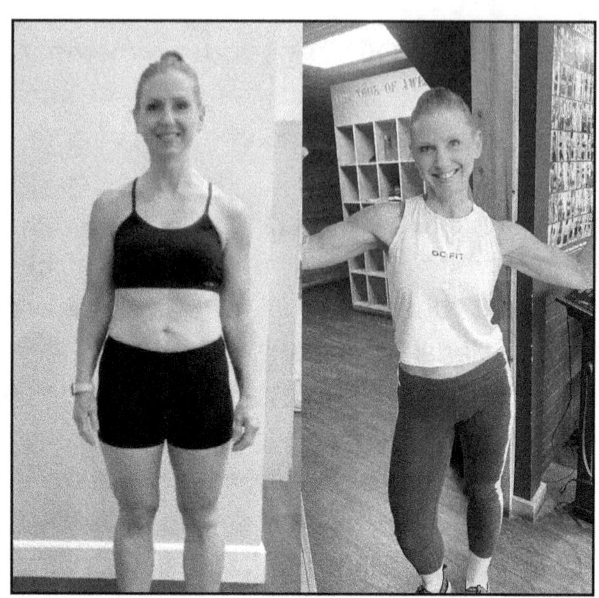

It's never too late, you're never too old, and staying hydrated with the Magic Fat Shed drink feels like a cravings-crushing superpower.

Look, this is a mindset book as much as a nutrition book. We are building you into the *who* so you can have, be, and look like the *what*. Just learning some new information isn't going to cut it. You already eat and drink things that you know you're not supposed to. You already consume things that aren't aligned with your conscience and cause you to have regret. You lie to yourself and say I'm going to start eating healthy—"Monday." You do this over and over again.

One of the biggest reasons for this is because you really haven't linked your nutrition to something of *higher value*. Something or someone that you refuse to let down, like your kids or your family. You're still doing it for yourself. And because it's "just you," you'll let yourself down, tell yourself lies, and negotiate over and over again.

So, while you are building that "mental muscle" of discipline and learning to consciously link your nutrition to a higher value, having fewer cravings can really help. That's where the Magic Fat-Shred Drink comes in.

Here's the formula for the Magic Fat-Shred Drink and a breakdown of each ingredient and what it does for your body:

1. Water (64 oz)—The Foundation of Fat Loss

Boosts metabolism—even mild dehydration slows metabolism. Hydration keeps fat-burning optimized.

Flushes out toxins—your body stores toxins in fat cells. Staying hydrated helps detoxification, making it easier to shed fat.

Prevents cravings—hunger is often dehydration in disguise. Drinking this keeps cravings in check.

Supports energy levels—when you're hydrated, you stay alert, focused, and ready to *crush* your workouts.

2. Apple Cider Vinegar (ACV; up to 1/4 cup)—The Metabolic Accelerator

Enhances fat burning—ACV helps activate adenosine monophosphate-activated protein kinase (AMPK), an enzyme that promotes fat breakdown while reducing fat storage.

Stabilizes blood sugar—prevents insulin spikes, keeping you in a fat-burning state longer.

Reduces cravings—ACV increases satiety, making you less likely to reach for junk.

Aids digestion—improves stomach acid production, helping you absorb nutrients more efficiently.

Balances electrolytes—contains potassium, which helps offset sodium retention and prevents bloating.

3. Cayenne Pepper—The Thermogenic Torch

Fires up metabolism—capsaicin, the active compound, increases calorie burn through thermogenesis.

Suppresses appetite—studies show cayenne reduces hunger and food intake.

Boosts circulation—helps transport oxygen and nutrients to muscles for better fat oxidation.

Improves digestion—stimulates digestive enzymes, promoting gut health and nutrient absorption.

4. Lemon Juice (Optional)—The Detoxifier

Aids liver function—your liver is your fat-burning powerhouse, and lemon juice supports detoxification.

Boosts vitamin C levels—an essential antioxidant that supports immune function and helps combat oxidative stress from training.

Alkalizes the body—despite being acidic, lemon juice promotes an alkaline environment, which reduces inflammation.

Enhances hydration—improves water absorption for better cellular hydration.

5. One serving of **flavored, low-sodium, sugar-free electrolytes** sweetened with stevia.

I use a brand called Ultima because it has just 55 mg of sodium, it's sweetened with stevia, and it tastes amazing.

How Much Magic Fat-Shred Should I Drink?

There are a lot of opinions about how much water to drink. It depends on your size, how much you sweat, and what you do. But I like to keep it simple. Here's what I recommend for my coaching clients.

General Guidelines:
Women 64–128 oz (approximately .5–1 gallon)
Men 128–192 oz (approximately 1–1.5 gallons)
This is what I typically drink on the days I don't do the sauna or hike. If I hike or do the sauna, I add a half gallon (total 1.5 gallons or 192 oz). If I do both—hike and sauna—and if it's hot, I sometimes add a gallon (total 2 gallons or 256 oz).

192 oz (1.5 gallons)—if you're feeling it, go for it.

256 oz (2 gallons)—this is the maximum I would recommend.

When Should I Drink My Magic Fat-Shred Drink?

The best time to drink your first half gallon is first thing in the morning. This will help control your cravings at the beginning of the day. You want to "stay ahead" of your thirst. If you wait too long, or get behind, it can take a while to catch back up, and you might have to deal with some pretty powerful cravings in the meantime.

After the first half gallon, drink the rest throughout the day. I typically don't like to finish too late because I end up having to get up to pee in the middle of the night.

Can I Drink the Magic Fat-Shred Drink While Fasting?

Yes! Not only does it help with not being hungry while fasting, it actually helps enhance the fat-burning effects of your fast.

ACCELERATOR #2—THE MAGIC 36-HOUR FAST

As I'm writing this, I'm doing a 36-Hour Fast. The Magic 36-Hour Fast is one of my favorite secret weapons for accelerating the results of burning straight fat.

This is *not* a substitute for the 3 Rules—it works *with* the 3 Rules to help you get leaner and healthier faster. It's also great for helping people who are diabetic or have prediabetes improve their insulin sensitivity.

It's important to note that you shouldn't do the Magic 36-Hour Fast more than one time per week. Any more than that and you'll have the *opposite effect* you're looking for by slowing your metabolism. I recommend to my coaching clients, if they *love it*, to do it once per week, and if they *like* it, to do it every two weeks until they're as lean as they want to be. Then, they can do it every once in a while for maintenance to get a "reset" effect.

I'm going to show you how to easily (for the most part) do a Magic 36-Hour Fast without feeling starved or hungry at all, while getting the best results and having energy. On average, my coaching clients lose 1 to 2 pounds of pure body fat after each 36-hour fast, and I have them do it every 1 to 2 weeks until they are as lean as they want to be. That's a lot of additional fat loss per month in addition to burning fat from following The 3. This has been my experience with more than 1,000 coaching clients, and I expect this every time, but my lawyer says I have to add that everyone is different and your results may vary.

The reason for the fat loss isn't just the fasting. It's the specific way I'm going to have you deplete your glycogen—the sugar stored in your cells—that will allow you to burn straight fat for energy.

Fat burning is awesome, but one of the best benefits is how it plays into creating *who* you are—yep, we're back to mindset. Even though I'm going to show you how to make the Magic 36-Hour Fast as easy as possible, at some point in your fast, it might be hard. It will expose the weaknesses in your mindset. You need to identify those weaknesses and destroy them.

You'll start to give yourself an out. Do not give in. You might tell yourself you *need* to eat. You don't. Shut up and keep going. You might even have some periods where you have legit hunger pains. *Good* because without pain, there can be no pleasure. The contrast is necessary to fully be in a grateful state.

There's also a certain alertness and clarity that only comes from fasting. The absence of food taps into our ancestral DNA and puts us in an elevated mindset. We go into hunting mode—sharper, clearer, more driven.

The only way to gain true confidence is by overcoming hard things and holding your word to yourself. The *pride* and *self-respect* that follows a 36-hour fast is extremely powerful. There's also a mental reset that happens by not eating for more than a day.

What do I mean by a mental reset? When you empty out your body with a Magic 36-Hour Fast, everything you ate before, good or bad, is gone by the end of it. Whether you decided to have a cheat day and your body is paying for it, or you've been following The 3 perfectly, you're going to feel better when you have a clean, blank whiteboard to start from. Since this whole thing is contingent on your mindset, this is a powerful tool.

HOW EXACTLY DO YOU DO THE MAGIC 36-HOUR FAST?

The Magic 36-Hour Fast is where you don't eat for 36 straight hours. For example, Wednesday at 8 p.m., you stop eating. Thursday you don't eat at all. Friday at 8 a.m. you start eating again.

Really, think of it as just one day without eating. Since in the example above, on Wednesday you stop eating at 8 at night, it's no big deal because that's close to when you would normally stop eating anyway. You'll get 5 to 9 hours of your fast in your sleep (depending on how much you sleep). Then, you just don't eat food Thursday. On Friday, you can break your fast at 8 in the morning.

This is just one way to do it. The important thing is to make sure you fast for 36 hours straight, no matter when you choose to start. If you stop eating at 6 p.m. on a Monday, for instance, then your fast will end at 6 a.m. on Wednesday. The number stays the same—just shift the time from p.m. to a.m. or vice versa.

The other important thing about scheduling your fast is to do it at a time when you'll be busy. I typically would never do my fasting on a weekend because I've got a lot more free time on my hands. Free time means giving my brain time to be bored enough to start thinking about food. Personally, I start my fast on a Thursday at 8 p.m., then I won't eat Friday, and then I break my fast on Saturday morning. But if I broke it on Sunday, and all day Saturday I was around my family and they were eating together and enjoying their meals, it would feel like I was missing out.

Benefits of the Magic 36-Hour Fast

1. Loss of body fat

You'll lose an average of 1 to 2 lbs of fat.

2. Reset of your insulin responsiveness

When you give your body a break from insulin for 36 hours, it becomes more insulin responsive or sensitive. This means that your body needs less insulin to get the same response. *Less insulin* equals *less fat storage*. This is also a very effective step to help prediabetic people get back into the normal range. I've had many type 2 diabetic coaching clients cure their diabetes faster by incorporating fasting when they follow The 3.

3. Mental clarity

Our ancestors were very focused on hunting and finding food when they didn't have food for a prolonged period of time. It's a survival mechanism built into our DNA that increases our drive and allows us to go to great lengths to find food. It helps cut out all the BS and distractions that don't really matter so we can have a singular purpose. Since in the 21st century, we aren't living in the jungle, that focus turns to business, family, and accomplishing goals. Life becomes simpler, and you're able to see more clearly the distractions and things that don't really matter for what they really are.

A lot of coaching clients have had so many bad experiences with nutrition that if they don't see results fast enough, they can get discouraged and quit. The Magic 36-Hour Fast is one of the most powerful results accelerators when you do it right, like we do with The 3.

My coaching client Natalie was one of those people who was inspired by seeing results quickly. So I had her do a 36-hour fast every week until she got to her desired leanness. Because of the system that I've invented for doing the Magic 36-Hour Fast when following The 3, not only are the *results accelerated*, but you're not hungry and you have a ton of *energy*, almost like having a *superpower*.

By following The 3 and adding the Magic 36-Hour Fasts, Natalie was able to see physical results so fast, she was hooked. I'll let Natalie tell you in her own words.

I've tried calorie counting in the past, but it was so hard to stay on track. I felt hungry all the time. Working with Steve was so easy, though. He always had a solution or a yummy recipe for me to try that made following The 3 fun, but the biggest game-changer for me was the Magic 36-Hour Fast.

Because I see results so fast, it's the perfect reset to keep me focused and give me that quick high. They're also great when you need to prepare for a special event—do them once a week for a month, and when the day comes, you'll feel beautiful and confident in yourself. Trust me, it's so much better than a diet pill.

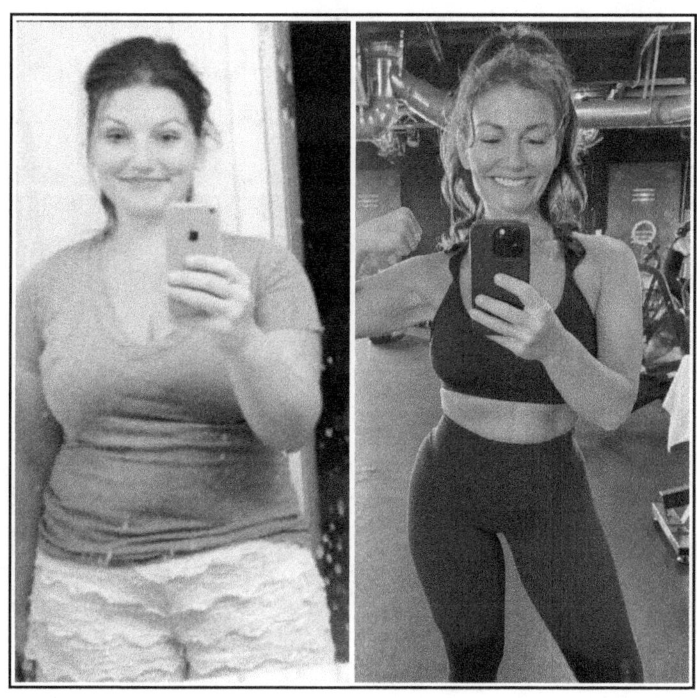

How You Will Feel During the Magic 36-Hour Fast

The way you feel is 95 percent determined by your attitude. If you make a huge deal of it and go into it complaining and saying "this is going to be so hard" and feeling sorry for yourself, you'll most likely have a difficult experience. Remember, we're creating you into the *who*, and then you'll look like the *what*.

You should go into this like anything you take on. Ask yourself, how would someone you admire do it? Think to yourself, "This is going to make me better in so many ways—leaner, mentally stronger, and more confident. I'm going to feel so proud." Go into this like a boss with a positive attitude, and you'll have a congruent experience. Go into it weak and negative, expecting it to suck, and it probably will.

Follow my exact instructions, and you'll love it. Here are some examples of what you can expect:

Most common responses
More energy
Clear-headedness
Focused
Alert
Positive
Hungry at times, but not sustained hunger

Less common responses
Anxious
Headache (usually if you don't follow all my instructions)
Extremely hungry (again, usually due to not following all my instructions)

What to Do If You Feel Awful

This is very rare (it happens less than 5 percent of the time) and in almost all cases, it's because people didn't follow my exact instructions. I have no idea why some people decide not to follow my instructions. I guess they just think they know better, or they select which of my instructions they think isn't that important to follow and don't bother—and they end up paying the price.

If this happens, and you really feel horrible, just resume eating, and try again in a week.

> **PRO TIP for Women:** There are hormonal conditions that can occur in females that can make the Magic 36-Hour Fast a bad idea. Sometimes it's predictable, and congruent with your cycle, other times it can be random. On the rare times when women feel awful during a Magic 36-Hour Fast, they often try to "tough it out." *Don't.* If it just doesn't *feel right*, please break your fast with your SCT meal and try again next week. This is *not* a reflection of your mental toughness, and it does *not* represent a failure. It's just a physiological circumstance that's beyond your control, and it's okay.

What You Can Eat/Drink

Eat:

No food at all. Don't try to outsmart this. Just do not eat.
No supplements

Drink:
Your best option—The Magic Fat-Shred Drink. See recipe on page 82.

Water

Green or black tea (be careful—some people feel nauseous if they drink tea on an empty stomach, so if you've never tried it, don't have the first time be during your 36-hour fast)

Black coffee (this *really* helps)

Sparkling water (I like to mix sparking water with some fresh lemon juice and liquid stevia. It tastes like sparking lemonade)

Carbonated zero calorie sodas that use 0 glycemic sweeteners like stevia (e.g., Zevia soda)

How to Prepare
I'm going to use the example of starting the Magic 36-Hour Fast Wednesday at 8 p.m. and breaking your fast Friday at 8 a.m. You don't need to use these days and times, I just like to do it in the middle of the week when I'm the busiest and can get the most benefit from the mental clarity aspect.

WEDNESDAY

It's very important to hydrate throughout the day. Remember, the same part of our brain that tells us we're hungry is also the part that signals that we're thirsty. Sometimes, those messages can get crossed. So, we might feel like we're very hungry when we're really just thirsty.

So, throughout the day, drink one to two gallons of the Magic Fat-Shred Drink. (Do not skip this step!)

Eat all your normal meals following the 3 Rules. Do *not* eat an SCT meal after your workout. We're trying to *deplete* glycogen, not *replace* it.

Prepare your hydro flasks with the Magic Fat-Shred Drink for the next day.

Stop eating at 8 p.m. (You may adjust this time depending on your schedule and lifestyle.)

THURSDAY

No eating!

Weigh yourself when you wake up (make a note).

I start my morning off with black coffee.

Try to get your first half gallon (64 oz) of the Magic Fat-Shred Drink as early as you can so you can stay ahead of your hunger. The ingredients in the Magic Fat-Shred Drink not only hydrate you but *drastically* reduce hunger. This is a must.

Now, we have to deplete as much glycogen, which is stored glucose in your muscles and cells, as possible so we can burn straight fat for energy tomorrow. Get in an hour-long, intense workout followed by 1 to 2 hours of steady-state cardio. I like to do HIIT (high-intensity interval training) workouts (a blend of short bursts of cardio and weightlifting—see www.steve-hochman.com for sample workouts). For the 1 to 2 hours of steady state, I typically either jump on a treadmill and walk on a slight incline while I watch Netflix or listen to a podcast, or go on a long walk or jog with my dog.

For the rest of the day, I like to stay busy and continue to drink the Magic Fat-Shred Drink, black coffee, and zero-calorie sodas like Zevia.

FRIDAY

The big pay off! Now that you're in a "glycogen-depleted state," it's time to *burn straight fat*!

Before you break your fast, weigh yourself and make a note.

If you started your fast at 8 p.m. Wednesday, then you'll break your fast at 8 a.m. today. You can go longer if you want.

Before you break your fast, now that you are in a "glycogen-depleted state" you MUST get a long workout in. Your body is primed and ready to use fat for fuel. This is the *most important* part!

The workout: my personal favorite is a 2-hour intense hike followed by 20 minutes in the sauna. You can do that, or a 1-hour HIIT workout followed by a 1- to 2-hour brisk walk or jog

Weigh yourself, then break your fast! You must break your fast with an SCT meal—carbs, protein, and no more than 5 grams of fat because the insulin spike will absorb the fat into your cells, and we want to avoid that. *Never* break your fast with a high-fat meal.

My favorite "break the fast" SCT meal is this:
1 to 2 cups fat free Greek yogurt
Mix in one scoop whey protein
Add 1 cup blueberries
2 medium red potatoes on the side.
For more SCT meals, go to www.stevehochman.com.

Some people have a sensitive stomach when they break their fast. If this is the case, have a cup of bone broth 15 minutes before your SCT. The bone broth will coat your stomach and get it prepared for your SCT meal.

Weigh yourself and make a note.

Wait 1.5 to 2 hours (so all the insulin is out of your bloodstream) then eat your normal meals (following Rules 1 and 2)

Saturday morning, right when you wake up, weigh yourself to see your net weight loss—the fat you actually lost, instead of weight loss just because you had less food in your body. I typically see my clients lose between 1 and 2 pounds of pure fat.

ACCELERATOR #3— INTERMITTENT FASTING

Intermittent fasting is different from the Magic 36-Hour Fast because it's shorter and can be done daily. Here's how it works: you fast (aka don't eat) for 16 hours followed by an 8-hour eating window. In other words, you eat all the food you would typically eat in a normal day, only it's compressed to within an 8-hour period. While you are fasting, no caloric intake is allowed (as little as 10 calories can break a fast). This can include many vitamins and supplements.

Here's a quick story about Matt, a coaching client who used intermittent fasting to accelerate his transformation.

To be honest, before 2024, I'd lost my connection with my overall fitness and sense of self. I'd tried so many "diets" over the years—macro-counting, calorie restrictions, low-carb, you name it. Every time I'd start strong, but eventually, I'd feel drained, frustrated, or restricted. None of it felt sustainable, and I'd always find myself back at square one. I wanted something different, something that wasn't just about food but about reclaiming who I am.

Then, I got an email from Steve inviting me to rejoin OC|FIT. The timing was right, so I jumped in. After I started working out again, Steve introduced me to his nutrition challenge. From day one, this approach was a GAME-CHANGER. His program wasn't a "diet" at all—it was a lifestyle shift that was easy to follow, practical, and designed for real, lasting results. Following his three rules under his mentorship, I didn't feel like I was depriving myself. It made sense in a way that all those other "diets" never did.

I felt like I could do more, though, so at the two-month point, Steve helped me incorporate intermittent fasting four times a week into my program. I started seeing results even faster, and before another month passed, I was shredded, with a visible six-pack and the best muscle definition of my life. It wasn't just about the pounds lost, though. I felt a renewed energy and confidence—like I was uncovering the person I wanted to be all along.

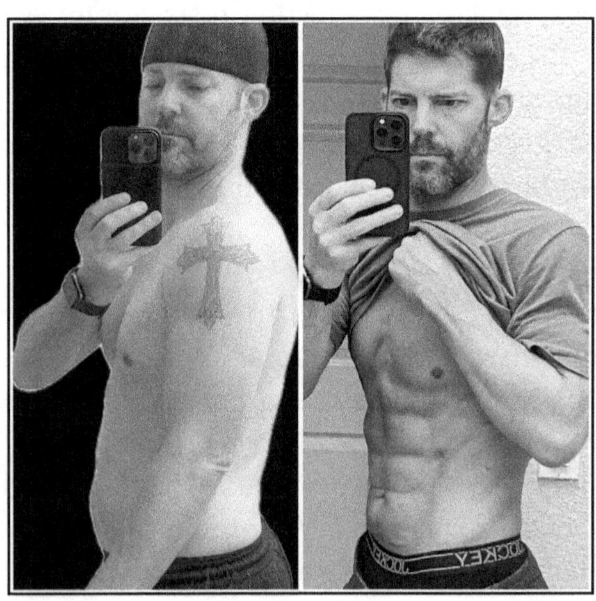

I need to stress that intermittent fasting is not a miracle solution or a way to get away with not following The 3. It just makes the results happen a little faster.

There are a few main reasons that I intermittent fast about four days per week. I have more energy and mental clarity in the morning and early afternoon while I'm fasting. I get a better workout, probably because the blood, oxygen, and energy that is not required for my digestive system is now available for my muscles and cardiovascular system. And, of course, it helps me to stay lean and mean all year round by helping my system be more efficient with insulin.

When you overuse anything in the human body, it becomes less effective, so when you get a 16-hour break from insulin, your body needs less of it to do its job, which results in less fat storage. That's why intermittent fasting is one of my accelerators for The 3.

Here are five more science-based benefits that you get with intermittent fasting:

1. **Lower pro-inflammatory cytokines:** intermittent fasting can decrease levels of proteins that promote inflammation, such as IL-6 and TNF-α.
2. **Reduced oxidative stress:** fasting helps lessen oxidative stress by decreasing the number of free radicals that can cause cellular damage, which contributes to reducing inflammation.
3. **Better gut health:** intermittent fasting can improve the balance of good and bad bacteria in the gut, which is significant for controlling inflammation and maintaining a healthy immune response.

4. **Reduced visceral fat:** intermittent fasting, when combined with The 3, speeds up weight loss, especially around the abdomen, which is linked to lower levels of chronic inflammation.

5. **Creation of hormonal adjustments that reduce inflammation:**

   Lower insulin: fasting helps your body produce less insulin. High insulin levels can cause inflammation, so reducing insulin helps prevent it.

   Boosted adiponectin: fasting increases a hormone called adiponectin, which lowers inflammation and improves your body's ability to handle insulin.

   Cortisol control: fasting helps keep cortisol, the stress hormone, at normal levels. Too much cortisol can lead to inflammation, so managing it helps reduce inflammation.

   Additional growth hormone: fasting raises levels of human growth hormone (HGH), which aids in tissue repair and reduces inflammation.

   Balanced hunger hormones: fasting helps regulate hormones like ghrelin and leptin, which control hunger and fullness. This balance helps prevent overeating and reduces inflammation related to excess weight.

PRO TIP: One of the biggest reasons people have a difficult time with intermittent fasting is because they're dehydrated. The hypothalamus sends signals of both hunger and thirst, and those signals can get confused for one another. Hydrate yourself before and during by drinking at least one gallon of the Magic Fat-Shred Drink for the best intermittent fasting experience.

WHAT TO EAT AND DRINK WHILE INTERMITTENT FASTING

The best case is to stay at zero calories. Stick to consuming the items listed below. A cup of black coffee, and a tablespoon of lemon juice has 2 to 3 calories, and that's acceptable; the rest of the items have zero calories.

Magic Fat-Shred Drink (a must)
Black coffee!!!! (liquid stevia optional)
Any herbal tea
Water
Lemon water (liquid stevia optional)
Noncaloric carbonated beverages (stevia optional)
Sparkling water

Example of Eating–Fasting Schedules

PRO TIP: To quickly calculate what time you break your 16-hour fast based on when you start your fast, just add 4 hours to when you start your fast. For example, if you start your fast at 8 p.m., just add 4 hours, so you'd break your fast at 12 p.m. the next day. Another example would be if you started your fast at 10 p.m., adding four hours to 10 p.m. would count out to 11, 12, 1, 2. So you'd break your fast at 2 p.m. the next day.

Example Schedule #1

Start eating at 1 p.m., stop eating at 9 p.m., and resume eating at 1 p.m. the next day.

If you stop eating at 9 p.m., go to bed at 10 p.m., and wake up at 6 a.m., 8 hours of your fast happens while you are sleeping—so just 8 more hours to go!

Other Examples of Eating Windows

Eat meals 9 a.m. to 5 p.m.
Eat meals 10 a.m. to 6 p.m.
Eat meals noon to 8 p.m.

For maximum fat burning, time your workouts so that you exercise fasted and break your 16-hour fast right after your workout. Since your body will release a higher-than-normal amount of insulin when you break your fast, be sure to break your fast with your Strategic Carb Timing (SCT) meal. As I explained earlier, this is a combination of glucose (fruit) and starch (for example, potato, rice) and protein that has no more than 5 grams of fat (like whey protein powder). *Remember*—have no more than 5 grams of fat when you break your fast, or you *will* absorb that fat.

Results of Working Out While Fasting

More energy (blood, oxygen, and energy are not being used for digestion)

More fat burning (when you deplete your stored glycogen, you begin to use fat as a fuel source)

I recommend you get over any thought that you are "weak" if you don't eat before a workout. When I first started intermittent fasting, I thought I would feel that way—like it would be a big deal. After a while, I forgot that I hadn't eaten before my workouts and realized I was actually having my best workouts while fasted.

Do not consume fat in the first meal after breaking your fast. Remember Rule 2: you automatically get an insulin spike when you break your fast that will cause you to absorb and store the fat you consume.

Try to time the breaking of your fast to right after your workout. (If that doesn't work with your schedule, it's okay.)

Here's how it works:

(Optimal) Time it so you finish your workout when it's time to break your fast. In this case, enjoy your SCT meal. Carbs, protein, and no more than 5 grams of fat.

Break your fast before workout. Just have protein and veggies, but no carbs and no more than 5 grams of fat.

My number-one meal to break my fast and the perfect post workout meal is as follows:

- 1 cup fat free Greek yogurt.
- 1 scoop whey protein
- 1 cup blueberries

Mix these together, then follow it with:

- 1 medium sweet or red potato
- No butter—you can add salt; I like Tajin seasoning

Sweet potato cooking instructions:

Oven—425°F for 40–50 min

Air fryer—370°F for 35–45 min

Microwave—5–12 minutes (but test first because each microwave is different)

To recap:

The Accelerators help kick your fitness, and especially your fat burning, into high gear.

- **Magic Fat-Shred Drink:** a specially formulated drink that hydrates, aids in fat mobilization, and curbs cravings. Shoot for 1 to 2 gallons a day.

Ingredients: cayenne pepper, apple cider vinegar, low-sodium electrolytes, and water (see recipe on p. 82).

- **36-Hour Fast:** 36 hours in which you don't eat, followed by an exercise routine that leads to increased fat burning and insulin sensitivity.
  You'll lose 1 to 2 pounds of fat per fast.
  Don't do it more than once per week.
  Keep your mindset positive—but if it feels awful, stop!
- **Intermittent fasting:** giving yourself an 8-hour eating window on the days you choose to intermittent fast—for me, around 4 days per week. This enhances the effects of the other accelerators.
  It improves your mental clarity and insulin efficiency.
  It also reduces pro-inflammatory cytokines and oxidative stress on your cells.

6

Eating Guidelines and Recipes

The power of The 3 goes far beyond just shutting down fat storage and being ultra healthy. The 3 makes eating healthy *fun*. Instead of having "cheat meals," you can now just switch out a couple of ingredients, turning them into fat-shred meals.

I've included some of my favorite recipes in this chapter. But I am creating *fresh new* recipes each week. To see how to get access to the entire library of the 3 Rule recipes, plus new ones weekly, head over to www.stevehochman.com.

Even though this isn't a calorie-reliant system, a lot of people want to know, "How often should I eat?" A good rule of thumb is every three hours from when you wake up to when you go to bed. I go into this in more detail in the food logs, but for example, you could do the following:

DAY ONE	DAY TWO	DAY THREE
6 a.m. breakfast	8 a.m. breakfast	5 a.m. early breakfast
9 a.m. snack	11 a.m. snack	8 a.m. breakfast
12 p.m. lunch	2 p.m. lunch	11 a.m. snack
3 p.m. snack	5 p.m. SCT meal	2 p.m. lunch
6 p.m. dinner	8 p.m. dinner	5 p.m. SCT meal
9 p.m. dessert		8 p.m. dinner

The important thing is that you don't just graze all day. There used to be this rumor that if you grazed all day on small things, you would force your metabolism to be in overdrive and burn more fat. *This is one of many myths that this book cuts through.* Scientific research actually shows that the opposite is true.

I've worked with people who will literally eat all day long—like every 10 minutes they're eating something. I've found that when I tell them to consolidate the exact same amount of food (all 3 Rule food, but the exact same amount of food) and allow two to three hours between meals, they get measurably better results.

Why do you burn more fat when you have two to three hours in between meals, versus if you eat the same amount of food but you never stop eating and graze all day? Here's the science behind it: every time you eat, especially carbohydrate-rich foods, your insulin levels rise to help process the glucose from the food. When your insulin is elevated, you burn less fat because the body prioritizes using the glucose from the food for energy. When you space your meals out, it gives your insulin levels time to return to baseline and your body shifts to burning fat for energy during those periods. Basically, when you're eating, you're storing fat. When you're not eating, you're using fat for energy.

I'm sure some of you are wondering, so let me start by saying this: I *do not* bake. I cook, grill, air fry, freeze, and microwave. This is not a baking book or traditional cookbook. I'm not into formulas, exact ingredient measurements, or exact oven temperatures. When things are too complicated, they don't get done. I have a family, a beautiful wife who's my best friend, and at the time of writing this book, three kids aged 18, 16, and 3; multiple businesses; hundreds of coaching clients; and my own workouts. Therefore, everything I make is quick and easy with few ingredients and loose measurements.

I'm listing a lot of brands that are my favorites in these recipes. I'm not necessarily affiliated with any of these brands. My program's always been just about me sharing what works for me. I'm a regular guy with regular genetics, not some anomaly who's lean no matter what. What works for me is what happens to work for just about everybody.

With that being said, brands change their formulas all the time. So even if I list something here, it's still your job to look it up and verify for yourself.

People say to me all the time, "I can't believe I can have this! It tastes so bad for you!" You're going to swear you're eating junk food, but the truth is you're giving yourself exactly what you need to be lean and healthy without the yo-yo effect of high glucose-releasing foods. My client Patty had this to say about it:

When I decided to join Steve's program, I was nervous. I worried it would be so restrictive that I'd just end up giving up again. But I was pleasantly surprised—this was nothing like what I'd done before. Week by week, I started seeing small but noticeable changes. For the first time, I felt like I was on a path I could actually stick with. The food was realistic and easy to make, the plan was simple, and with Steve's encouragement I started feeling more motivated than ever.

By the end of the 6 weeks, I couldn't believe my own transformation. I fit into my skinny jeans again, but more than that, I had gained back my confidence. What started as a program turned into a lifestyle that I actually enjoy. Life feels amazing now. I have energy, I feel strong, and I'm proud of

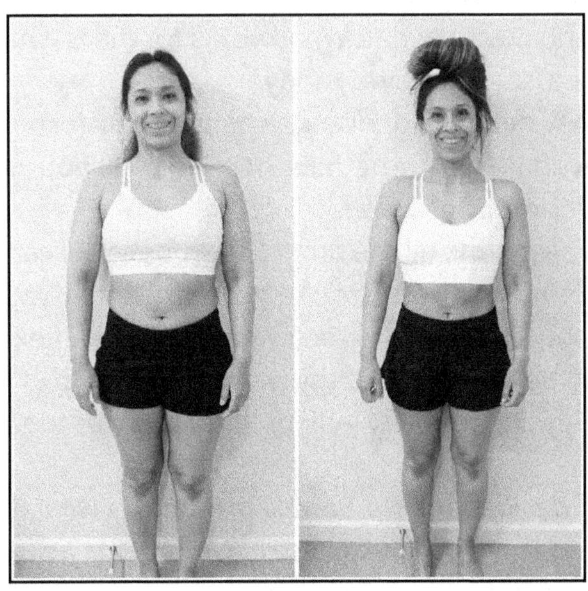

The information in this book will act as your shield against a mountain of food industry *misinformation* and *disinformation*. Put a food you're interested in through the filter of The 3, and 99 percent of the time, you'll be protected from the bad stuff that companies try to sneak into your body. But, as I noted earlier, be aware that sometimes food companies change their ingredients over time. Sometimes, it's because they want a cheaper ingredient so they can make more net profit, or maybe they were bought by a bigger company that knows which ingredients are the most addictive. Usually, the ingredients they change break Rule 1: Stay Under 25 on the glycemic index (GI). So, even if I list a specific brand, it's still your responsibility to check the ingredients yourself.

The recipes in this chapter are just guidelines. You may change, add, or subtract ingredients. I *encourage* this. That's the whole point of learning The 3—so that you have the ability to apply the rules and make your own creations. For any recipe (except your Strategic Carb Timing [SCT] meal), as long as you keep all ingredients under 25 on the GI, you're good! So, use these recipes to get you started and inspire you to create your own favorite meals! You can also check out www.stevehochman.com for more recipes.

SCT RECIPES

---

1. Berry Bliss Protein Bowl

Ingredients:
- 1 cup fat-free Greek yogurt
- 1 scoop vanilla whey protein
- ½ cup mixed berries (blueberries, raspberries, strawberries)

Instructions:
1. Mix protein powder into Greek yogurt until smooth.
2. Top with mixed berries.
3. Serve immediately.

2. Post-Workout Sweet Potato Mash

Ingredients:
- 1 medium-sized sweet potato, cooked
- 1 scoop vanilla or chocolate whey protein powder
- ½ cup almond milk

Instructions:
1. Mash the cooked sweet potato in a bowl.
2. Mix in whey protein and almond milk until smooth.
3. Serve warm or chilled.

3. Tropical Recovery Smoothie

Ingredients:
- 1 scoop whey protein (vanilla or tropical flavor)
- ½ cup pineapple chunks
- ½ cup mango chunks
- 1 cup unsweetened almond milk
- Ice cubes

Instructions:
1. Blend all ingredients in a blender until smooth.
2. Serve immediately.

4. Lean Chicken & Rice Delight

Ingredients:

- 4 oz grilled chicken breast
- ½ cup cooked white rice
- 1 tsp lime juice
- 1 tbsp chopped cilantro

Instructions:

1. Combine chicken and rice on a plate.
2. Drizzle lime juice and sprinkle with cilantro.
3. Serve warm.

5. Banana Oat Protein Pancakes

Ingredients:

- ½ cup rolled oats
- 1 scoop vanilla whey protein powder
- 1 medium banana, mashed
- 1 egg white

Instructions:

1. Mix all ingredients into a batter.
2. Heat a nonstick skillet and pour batter to form pancakes.
3. Cook until golden brown on both sides.

6. Strawberry Shortcake Protein Parfait

Ingredients:

- 1 cup fat-free Greek yogurt
- 1 scoop vanilla whey protein powder
- ½ cup sliced strawberries
- ¼ cup crushed low-GI granola (optional)

Instructions:

1. Mix protein powder into yogurt.
2. Layer yogurt mixture, strawberries, and granola in a glass.
3. Repeat layers and serve chilled.

---

7. Cinnamon Apple Protein Oats

Ingredients:

- ½ cup rolled oats
- 1 small apple, diced
- 1 scoop cinnamon-flavored protein powder
- 1 tsp ground cinnamon

Instructions:

1. Cook oats according to package instructions.
2. Stir in diced apple, protein powder, and cinnamon.
3. Serve warm.

8. Muscle Recovery Pasta Bowl

Ingredients:
- 1 cup cooked whole wheat or brown rice pasta
- 4 oz grilled chicken breast
- ½ cup no-sugar-added marinara sauce

Instructions:
1. Combine pasta, chicken, and marinara sauce in a bowl.
2. Heat until warm and serve.

9. Pineapple Chicken Rice Bowl

Ingredients:
- ½ cup cooked white rice
- 4 oz grilled chicken breast
- ¼ cup pineapple chunks
- 1 tsp soy sauce or coconut aminos
-

Instructions:
1. Combine rice, chicken, and pineapple in a bowl.
2. Drizzle with soy sauce and mix well.

10. Peachy Protein Smoothie

Ingredients:
- 1 scoop vanilla whey protein powder
- 1 medium peach, sliced
- 1 cup unsweetened almond milk
- Ice cubes

Instructions:
1. Blend all ingredients in a blender until smooth.
2. Serve immediately.

DESSERTS

1. Fat-Shred Gooey Chocolate Chip Cookies

Ingredients:
- 2 cups almond flour
- ½ cup monk fruit sweetener
- 2 tbsp coconut oil
- 1 tbsp vanilla extract
- 1 tsp baking powder
- 2 eggs
- Lily's sugar-free chocolate chips (as much as desired)

Instructions:
1. Preheat your oven to 350°F (175°C). Line a baking sheet with parchment paper.
2. In a large bowl, combine almond flour, monk fruit sweetener, coconut oil, vanilla extract, baking powder, and eggs. Mix until a smooth cookie dough forms.
3. Fold in Lily's sugar-free chocolate chips. Add as many as you'd like for extra gooeyness!

4. Scoop small amounts of the dough and place them on the prepared cookie sheet, spacing them evenly.
5. Bake for 12–18 minutes, depending on the thickness of the cookies. The edges should turn golden brown when done.
6. Allow cookies to cool on the baking sheet for 5–10 minutes before transferring them to a wire rack. Enjoy!

PRO TIPS:

For chewier cookies, bake on the shorter end of the time range.

Store in an airtight container at room temperature for up to three days or in the refrigerator for up to a week.

2. Fat-Shred Cheesecake with Chocolate Drizzle

(Makes 10–12 slices)

Ingredients

- Cheesecake Filling:
- 24 oz cream cheese (bring to room temp)
- 2 cups nonfat Greek yogurt
- 2½ tsp pure vanilla extract
- 1 tsp lemon juice
- 2/3 cup monk fruit
- ¼ cup almond flour

Crust:

- Cinnamon to taste
- 2 cups almond flour
- 4–6 tbsp butter

Instructions

Preheat oven to 350°F (175°C).

For the crust:

1. Combine all ingredients, pour into a lined 8- or 9-inch springform pan, press down evenly. Set aside while making the filling.
2. Fill any baking pan about halfway up with water, and place it on the oven's lower rack.
3. Beat all ingredients in a blender or food processor until just smooth (overbeating can cause cracking as it bakes).
4. Spread filling on top of prepared crust.
5. Place on the middle rack (above the rack with the water pan). Bake for 30 minutes (or 38 minutes if using an 8-inch pan), and do not open the oven at all during this time.
6. Once time is up, still do not open the oven, but turn off the heat and let the cheesecake sit in the oven an additional 5 minutes.
7. Remove from the oven—it will still look underdone.
8. Let cool on the counter 20 minutes.

9. Refrigerate overnight, during which time it will firm up considerably. I like to drizzle NuNaturals sugar-free chocolate syrup on top.

---

3. 3-Rule Fudge Chocolate Chip Brownies

Ingredients:
- 1 cup almond flour
- ½ cup unsweetened cocoa powder
- ½ tsp baking soda
- ¼ tsp sea salt
- 2 large eggs
- ½ cup unsweetened almond milk
- ½ cup granulated monk fruit sweetener
- 1 tsp vanilla extract
- ⅓ cup melted coconut oil or butter (grass-fed, optional)
- ½ cup Lily's sugar-free chocolate chips

Instructions:
1. Preheat your oven to 350°F (175°C). Line an 8 x 8-inch baking pan with parchment paper or grease it lightly with coconut oil.
2. Mix Dry Ingredients: In a medium bowl, whisk together almond flour, cocoa powder, baking soda, and sea salt.
3. Mix Wet Ingredients: In another bowl, beat eggs, almond milk, monk fruit sweetener, vanilla extract, and melted coconut oil (if using) until smooth.
4. Gradually add the dry ingredients into the wet mixture. Stir until well combined and smooth.
5. Fold in Lily's sugar-free chocolate chips.
6. Pour the batter into the prepared baking pan and spread evenly. Bake for 18 to 22 minutes or until a toothpick inserted in the center comes out with a few moist crumbs (not wet batter).
7. Let the brownies cool completely in the pan before slicing. Serve and enjoy!

PRO TIPS:

For a fudgier texture, underbake slightly and refrigerate after cooling.

Store leftovers in an airtight container in the refrigerator for up to five days.

Optional: Top with a drizzle of melted sugar-free chocolate or a dollop of fat-free Greek yogurt for an extra treat!

---

4. Chocolate Lava Cake

This is one of my go-to desserts to crush cravings while increasing your health and getting lean AF💪🏆.

Ingredients:

- 1 egg
- 1 scoop whey protein (I use strawberry flavored)
- ⅓ cup almond flour
- Lily's sugar-free dark chocolate chips
- NuNaturals (sugar-free) chocolate syrup

Instructions:

1. Add the following in a small bowl, then mix:
   - 1 egg
   - 1 scoop whey protein
   - ⅓ cup almond flour
   - ¼ cup Lily's sugar-free chocolate chips
2. Mix until thick and smooth
3. Microwave for 20 to 30 seconds (*do not overcook*)
4. It should be gooey and slightly hard on the edges.

5. Remove from the microwave and add NuNaturals chocolate syrup, some more sugar free chocolate chips ... (I also add a little peanut butter)

---

5. Cottage Cheesecake (Chocolate Chip/Chocolate Drizzle Optional)

Ingredients:

- 1 cup cottage cheese
- 1 scoop protein powder (vanilla or chocolate)
- Lily's sugar-free chocolate chips or drizzle

Instructions:

1. Blend cottage cheese with protein powder until smooth.
2. Top with Lily's sugar-free chocolate chips or drizzle.
3. Serve chilled.

---

6. Peanut Butter with Chocolate Chips

Ingredients:

- 1 tbsp natural peanut butter
- 1 tbsp Lily's sugar-free chocolate chips

Instructions:

1. Mix peanut butter and chocolate chips together.
2. Freeze for 10 minutes for a quick treat.

---

7. Protein Pudding

Ingredients:
- 1 scoop protein powder
- Splash of unsweetened almond milk
- 1 tsp vanilla extract
- ¼ cup Lily's sugar-free chocolate chips (optional)

Instructions:
1. Mix protein powder with a small amount of almond milk to form a thick consistency.
2. Stir in vanilla extract and Lily's sugar-free chocolate chips (if desired).
3. Chill before serving.

BREAKFASTS

---

1. Waffles (with Maple Syrup)

Ingredients:
- 1 cup almond flour
- 1 pinch of salt
- 1 tsp baking soda
- 4 eggs
- ¼ cup monk fruit sweetener
- 1 tsp vanilla extract
- 2 tbsp Lily's sugar-free chocolate chips (optional)

Instructions:
1. Preheat waffle iron.
2. Combine almond flour, salt, and baking soda in a large bowl.
3. In a separate bowl, whisk eggs, monk fruit, and vanilla extract.
4. Stir flour mixture into egg mixture (add Lily's sugar-free chocolate chips if desired).
5. Grease waffle iron.
6. Spoon batter onto hot waffle iron. Cook until golden.

2. Bacon Steak Eggs

Ingredients:

- 2 strips of bacon
- 4 oz steak
- 2 eggs

Instructions:

1. Cook bacon and steak in a skillet.
2. Fry eggs in the bacon grease.
3. Serve together for a hearty breakfast.

3. Pancakes with Maple Syrup

Ingredients:

- ½ cup rolled oats
- 1 medium banana
- 1 scoop vanilla whey protein powder
- 2 egg whites

Instructions:

1. Blend all ingredients into a batter.
2. Pour onto a greased skillet and cook each side until golden.
3. Top with sugar-free maple syrup.

4. Eggs, Rao's, and Mayo Scramble

Ingredients:
- 4 eggs
- 2 tbsp Rao's Marinara Sauce
- 1 tbsp mayonnaise (Ensure the mayonnaise complies with the 3 Rule guidelines.)

Instructions:
1. Scramble eggs in a skillet.
2. Mix in Rao's marinara sauce and mayonnaise before serving.

5. Cottage Cheese (I prefer low-fat Good Culture brand)

6. Cottage Cheese with Strawberry/Vanilla Protein

Ingredients:
- 1 cup cottage cheese
- 1 scoop strawberry or vanilla whey protein powder

Instructions:
Mix protein powder into cottage cheese until smooth.

7. Cottage Cheese Strawberry/Vanilla Protein with Lily's Sugar-Free Chocolate Chips

Ingredients:

- 1 cup cottage cheese
- 1 scoop protein powder (strawberry or vanilla)
- 2 tbsp Lily's sugar-free chocolate chips

Instructions:

1. Mix protein powder into cottage cheese.
2. Sprinkle with Lily's sugar-free chocolate chips.

8. 3-Ingredient Protein Chicken Strips

Ingredients:

- 1 lb shredded chicken
- 2 eggs
- 1 cup low-fat shredded cheese

Instructions:

1. Mix all ingredients in a bowl.
2. Season to taste.
3. Bake at 400°F for 20 minutes or air fry at 400°F for 10 minutes.

9. No Carb Bread Rolls

Ingredients:
- 2 cups almond flour
- 2 cups fat-free Greek yogurt
- Butter (optional)

Instructions:
1. Mix almond flour and Greek yogurt.
2. Form into rolls. Place butter in the center (optional).
3. Air fry at 350°F for 12 minutes, flip, and air fry for 3 more minutes.

10. Egg Muffins

Ingredients:
- 12 cups liquid egg whites or whole eggs
- Rao's Marinara Sauce (or any brand of marinara that is sugar and starch free)
- Favorite veggies (optional)
- Cooked ground beef (optional)

Instructions:
1. Mix sauce with liquid egg whites.
2. Spray muffin tin with coconut oil spray.
3. Fill with egg mixture. Bake at 350°F for 25 minutes.
4. Cool and store in refrigerator or freezer for later use.

11. Veggie Egg Scramble

Ingredients:

- 1–2 cups liquid egg whites (or 2–6 whole eggs)
- Chopped vegetables
- Rao's Marinara Sauce (optional)
- Salt and pepper
- Shredded cheese (optional)

Instructions:

1. Sauté or air fry vegetables with coconut oil until tender.
2. Add egg whites or whole eggs, cook until set.
3. Top with marinara or shredded cheese if desired.

LUNCHES AND DINNERS

1. Fat-Shred Nachos

Ingredients:

- Pork rinds (Always check ingredients!)
- Ground beef (grass-fed, cooked)
- Cheese (organic, no starch added)
- Buffalo sauce

Instructions:

1. Top pork rinds with ground beef, cheese, and sauce.
2. Microwave or bake to melt cheese.

2. Fat-Shred Tuna Sushi Rolls

Ingredients:

- 1 can tuna (packed in water, drained)
- 1–2 tbsp mayonnaise (Primal Kitchen or any brand with no sugar or starch)
- ½ avocado, sliced
- ½ cucumber, peeled and sliced
- Nori seaweed sheets (check for no added sugar)

Instructions:

1. Drain the tuna and mix it with mayonnaise in a small bowl until evenly combined. Ensure the mayonnaise complies with the 3 Rule guidelines.
2. Lay a sheet of nori seaweed on a flat surface or sushi rolling mat, with the shiny side facing down.
3. Spread the tuna mixture evenly across the bottom third of the nori.
4. Layer avocado slices and cucumber on top of the tuna.
5. Gently roll the nori tightly around the fillings. If needed, wet the edge of the nori with water to seal it securely.
6. Use a sharp knife to cut the roll into bite-sized pieces. Serve immediately and enjoy!

PRO TIPS:

Avoid adding any sauces or toppings with a glycemic index over 25.

Coconut aminos can be used as a dipping sauce if desired (check the label for 3 Rule compliance).

---

3. Fat-Shred Spicy Salmon Cut Roll

Shred fat with spicy salmon cut rolls🏆!!

Ingredients:
- Canned salmon
- Primal Kitchen Buffalo Ranch dressing
- Nori seaweed
- Cucumber
- Avocado
- Optional: Sushi roller (I got mine on Amazon for under five dollars)

Instructions:
1. Mash up the canned salmon with the Primal Kitchen Buffalo Ranch.
2. Across the end of the seaweed sheet, add a strip of avocado and cucumber rolled up with your sushi roller.
3. Cut the roll with a sharp knife and enjoy!

---

4. Air-Fried Chicken Nuggets (3 Rule Style)

Ingredients:
- 10 oz cooked chicken
- 1 egg
- 4 tbsp mozzarella cheese
- Optional seasonings: garlic powder, cayenne pepper, black pepper

Instructions:
1. Preheat air fryer to 400°F.
2. Shred cooked chicken.
3. Mix chicken, cheese, and egg in a bowl.
4. Form into nugget shapes and place on parchment paper.
5. Air fry for 10 minutes, flipping halfway.

5. Fat-Shred Air-Fried Chicken Tenders

Ingredients:
- 1 lb chicken tenders
- 1–2 eggs, beaten
- 1 cup almond flour
- 1 tbsp paprika
- 1 tbsp garlic powder
- Salt and pepper

Instructions:
1. Preheat air fryer to 400°F.
2. Pat chicken tenders dry.
3. Dip tenders into beaten eggs, then coat with almond flour mixture.
4. Air fry for 12 minutes, flipping halfway.

6. Air-Fried Veggies

Ingredients:
- Vegetables (e.g., brussels sprouts, broccoli, cauliflower, asparagus)
- Olive, avocado, or coconut oil spray
- Garlic powder or other seasonings (optional)

Instructions:
1. Prehat air fryer to 380°F.
2. Spray veggies with oil and season.
3. Air fry for 10–13 minutes, stirring halfway.

7. Crockpot Chicken

Ingredients:
- 4–8 organic chicken breasts
- 1 chopped yellow onion
- 4 cups spinach or kale
- 2 chopped bell peppers
- 2 cups chopped celery
- 1.5 jars Rao's Marinara Sauce

Instructions:
1. Add all ingredients to crockpot.
2. Cook on high for 4–6 hours.

8. Air-Fryer Carb-Less Pizza

Ingredients:
- Outer Isle Cauliflower Sandwich Thins
- Rao's no-sugar pasta sauce
- Shredded mozzarella cheese
- Garlic powder
- Oregano

Instructions:
1. Spread sauce, cheese, and seasonings on cauliflower thin.
2. Air fry at 400°F for 6 minutes.

---

9. Air-Fried Garlic Bread

Ingredients:
- Outer Isle Cauliflower Sandwich Thins
- Ghee butter spray
- Garlic powder
- Shredded parmesan cheese

Instructions:
3. Spread butter and seasonings on cauliflower thin.
4. Air fry at 400°F for 6 minutes.

---

10. Air-Fried Chicken Breast and Thighs

Ingredients:
- 4 medium chicken breast fillets or thighs (4–6 oz each)
- 1 tbsp olive oil
- 1 tsp smoked paprika
- 1 tsp cumin
- 1 tsp onion powder
- ½ tsp salt

Instructions:
1. Preheat air fryer to 400°F.
2. Coat chicken with oil and seasonings.
3. Air fry for 4 minutes per side or until internal temperature is 165°F.

11. Air-Fried Burgers

Ingredients:
*   1 lb ground beef (80 lean/20 fat mix)
*   ½ tsp salt
*   ½ tsp garlic powder
*   ½ tsp onion powder
*   ¼ tsp black pepper
*   Outer Isle Cauliflower Sandwich Thins

Instructions:
4. Combine beef and seasonings, then form patties.
5. Air fry at 360°F for 7 minutes per side.
6. Serve on cauliflower thins with toppings.

12. Air-Fried Steak

Ingredients:
*   1–2 steaks (e.g., Ribeye, NY Strip, or Tri-Tip, 1-inch thick)
*   1 tbsp olive oil
*   1 tsp Italian seasoning
*   Salt and pepper

Instructions:
1. Preheat air fryer to 400°F.
2. Rub steaks with oil and seasonings.
3. Air fry for 6 minutes per side for medium doneness.

13. Air-Fried Salmon

Ingredients:
- 4 salmon fillets
- 1 tbsp olive oil
- 1 tsp garlic powder
- ½ tsp paprika
- Salt and pepper

Instructions:
1. Preheat air fryer to 400°F.
2. Rub salmon with oil and seasonings.
3. Air fry for 7–9 minutes.

14. Creamy Chicken (or Tuna) Salad

Ingredients:
- Chopped organic chicken (or tuna in water)
- Lettuce
- Mayonnaise (Primal Kitchen or homemade)
- Rice vinegar
- Olive oil
- Optional toppings: olives, bell peppers, tomatoes

Instructions:
1. Mix mayonnaise, vinegar, and oil with chicken.
2. Toss with lettuce and toppings.

---

15. Hot Dogs

Ingredients:
- Outer Isle Cauliflower Sandwich Thins
- Organic chicken sausage or grass-fed beef hot dog
- Toppings: Primal Kitchen ketchup, mustard, pickles

Instructions:
1. Cook sausage or hot dog.
2. Serve on cauliflower thins with desired toppings.

---

16. Turkey or Roast Beef Sandwich

Ingredients:
- Outer Isle Cauliflower Sandwich Thins
- Turkey or roast beef (no sugar or starch added)
- Optional toppings: cheese, mustard, avocado, pickles, onions

Instructions:
1. Layer ingredients on cauliflower thins.
2. Serve as a sandwich.

17. Mexican Zucchini Boats

Ingredients:
- Zucchini
- Bell peppers
- Organic ground turkey
- Organic cheese
- Salsa verde

Instructions:
3. Preheat oven to 375°F. Cut zucchini in half and scoop out centers.
4. Roast zucchini for 25 minutes.
5. Cook turkey and peppers, add salsa verde.
6. Fill zucchini with turkey mixture, top with cheese, and bake for 15 more minutes.

18. Chicken Noodle Soup

Ingredients:
- 2 tbsp olive oil
- 1 cup celery, sliced thin
- 1 cup onion, chopped
- 2 garlic cloves, minced
- 8 cups chicken bone broth
- 2 bay leaves
- ½ tsp dried thyme
- ½ tsp dried oregano
- 1 package Miracle Noodles brand plant-based noodles
- 2 cups shredded organic chicken

7.

Instructions:
1. Sauté celery, onion, and garlic in olive oil.
2. Add broth, bay leaves, thyme, and oregano. Simmer for 10 minutes.
3. Add rinsed Miracle Noodles and chicken, then cook until heated.

Recipes Without Instructions:

19. Low Carb Chili

20. Spaghetti

21. Rigatoni (Red Lentil Pasta)

22. "Mac and Cheese" (Red Lentil Pasta)

23. No-Carb Enchilada Bake

24. Turkey Honey Mustard Panini

25. Pad Thai

SNACKS

1. Jicama

If you want the flavor to smack you in the face, add lemon juice and Tajin or chili powder.

2. Pork Rinds

(Always check ingredients! I use Epic brand or 4505, but only the Sea Salt ones because the other flavors have sugar.)

3. Cottage Cheese

4. I prefer low-fat, and my favorite brand by far is Good Culture.

4. Cottage Cheesecake (Chocolate Chip/Chocolate Drizzle Optional)

Ingredients:
- 1 cup cottage cheese
- 1 scoop protein powder (vanilla or chocolate)
- Lily's sugar-free chocolate chips or drizzle

Instructions:
1. Blend cottage cheese with protein powder until smooth.
2. Top with Lily's sugar-free chocolate chips or drizzle.
3. Serve chilled.

5. Fat-Free Greek Yogurt with Protein

Ingredients:
- 1 cup fat-free Greek yogurt
- 1 scoop whey protein powder (flavor of choice)

Instructions:
1. Mix protein powder into yogurt until smooth.
2. Serve immediately.

7. Celery with (or Without) Peanut Butter

Ingredients:
*   Celery sticks
*   1 tbsp natural peanut butter

Instructions:
Spread peanut butter onto celery sticks.

---

8. Celery with Organicville Ranch Dressing

Ingredients:
*   Celery sticks
*   Organicville Ranch dressing

Instructions:
Dip celery sticks into Organicville Ranch dressing.

---

9. Cauliflower Thin Garlic Bread

Ingredients:
*   Outer Isle Cauliflower Sandwich Thins
*   Olive oil spray
*   Garlic powder
*   Shredded parmesan cheese

Instructions:
1. Spray cauliflower thins with olive oil.
2. Sprinkle garlic powder and parmesan cheese on top.
3. Air fry at 400°F for 6 minutes.

**10. Seaweed Snacks

There should only be 3 ingredients: Seaweed, olive oil, and sea salt.

---

11. Rolled Turkey with Mustard, Primal Kitchen Buffalo Ranch, or Organicville Ranch

Ingredients:

- Turkey slices (check all ingredients—all must be 3-Rule approved)
- Mustard, Primal Kitchen Buffalo Ranch, or Organicville Ranch** (optional)

Instructions:

1. Spread chosen condiment onto turkey slices.
2. Roll into bite-sized wraps.

---

12. Rolled Roast Beef with Mustard, Buffalo Ranch, or Organicville Ranch

Ingredients:

- Slices of roast beef (check all ingredients—all must be 3-Rule approved)
- Mustard, Primal Kitchen Buffalo Ranch, or Organicville Ranch** (optional)

Instructions:

1. Spread chosen condiment onto roast beef slices.
2. Roll into bite-sized wraps.

13. Cauliflower Pizza

Ingredients:
- Outer Isle Cauliflower Sandwich Thins
- Rao's no-sugar pasta sauce
- Organic shredded mozzarella cheese
- Garlic powder and oregano

Instructions:
1. Spread sauce on cauliflower thin.
2. Sprinkle with cheese, garlic powder, and oregano.
3. Air fry at 400°F for 6 minutes.

14. Sugar-Free Chocolate Chips

1. (Keep in freezer for a cold treat)
2. My favorite brand is Lily's sugar-free dark chocolate chips

15. Egg Muffins

Ingredients:
- 1–2 cups liquid egg whites or whole eggs
- Rao's marinara sauce (or any sugar-free marinara)
- Favorite veggies (optional)
- Cooked ground beef (optional)

Instructions:
1. Mix marinara with egg whites or whole eggs.
2. Spray muffin tin with coconut oil spray.
3. Pour mixture into tin and bake at 350°F for 25 minutes.
4. Cool and store in fridge or freezer.

---

16. Air-Fried Bell Peppers

Ingredients:
- Bell peppers, chopped into 1- to 2-inch pieces
- Olive oil spray
- Tajin seasoning

Instructions:
1. Toss chopped bell peppers with olive oil and Tajin seasoning.
2. Air fry at 400°F for 11 to 13 minutes, stirring halfway.

DRINKS AND BEVERAGES

---

1. **Zevia Drinks**

These drinks taste like soft drinks but use a natural sweetener, so there is zero sugar. Popular flavors include Dr. Zevia and Ginger Root Beer.

---

2. **La Croix Drinks**

These are carbonated unsweetened drinks with natural flavor essences. You can drink them as-is or add a few drops of liquid stevia for sweetness.

---

3. **Waterloo Drinks**

Similar to La Croix, these are carbonated unsweetened drinks with natural flavor essences. Drink as-is or add liquid stevia.

---

4. **Tejava**

A high-quality unsweetened black tea that comes in a glass bottle.

---

5. **Coffee**

Hot or iced black coffee, hot or iced Americano, or cold brew. If you want to add something, use liquid stevia and/or unsweetened almond or cashew milk.

---

6. **Latte**

- 2 shots espresso (or a cup of coffee)
- ½ cup steamed or frothed unsweetened almond milk

Tip: Almond milk from the refrigerated section froths better than shelf-stable versions.

---

7. **Lemonade**

- Water
- Freshly squeezed lemon juice
- Liquid stevia (amount varies based on taste)

---

8. **Any Green, Black, or Yerba Mate Unsweetened Tea**

3. Serve hot or cold. Sweeten with liquid stevia if desired.

---

9. **Magic Fat-Shred Drink**

Ingredients:
- 16 oz cold water
- Juice from 1 lime
- 1 tbsp apple cider vinegar
- 1 tsp chia seeds
- 1–2 drops liquid stevia

Instructions:
1. Mix all ingredients and let sit for 5 to 10 minutes so chia seeds can expand.
2. Serve cold.

DRESSINGS/SAUCES

---

1. Apple Cider Vinaigrette

Ingredients:
- ¾ cup olive oil
- ¼ cup apple cider vinegar
- 2 tsp mustard
- ¼ tsp ground pepper
- ¼ tsp paprika
- ⅛ tsp sea salt
- ⅛ tsp garlic powder
- Liquid stevia (optional)

Instructions:
1. Combine all ingredients in a bowl or jar.
2. Whisk or shake well before serving.

2. Balsamic Vinaigrette

Ingredients:
- ½ cup apple cider vinegar
- ½ cup balsamic vinegar
- 2 tbsp water
- ⅔ cup olive oil
- ½ tsp dried basil
- ½ tsp garlic powder
- ½ tsp onion powder
- ½ tsp dried oregano
- 1 tsp sea salt
- Liquid stevia (optional)

Instructions:
1. Mix all ingredients in a jar or bottle.
2. Shake well before serving.

3. Thousand Island Dressing

Ingredients:
- 1 cup mayonnaise (Primal Kitchen or homemade)
- 2 tbsp sugar-free ketchup
- 1 tbsp apple cider vinegar
- ½ tsp paprika
- Salt and pepper to taste

Instructions:
1. Mix all ingredients in a bowl until smooth.
2. Adjust seasoning to taste.

4. Creamy Honey Mustard

Ingredients:
- 1 cup mayonnaise (Primal Kitchen or homemade)
- 2 tbsp Dijon mustard
- 1 tbsp liquid stevia or honey (if not strictly following the glycemic index rule)
- 1 tsp apple cider vinegar

Instructions:
1. Whisk all ingredients in a bowl until creamy.
2. Store in the refrigerator until ready to use.

---

5. Creamy Marinara

Ingredients:
- 1 cup Rao's Marinara Sauce
- ¼ cup heavy cream (optional)
- 1 tbsp olive oil

Instructions:
1. Heat marinara sauce in a saucepan over medium heat.
2. Stir in heavy cream and olive oil.
3. Simmer until warm and creamy.

EATING OUT

PRO TIP: I always recommend making your own food as much as possible, but when you go out, be sure to look up or ask about all ingredients to make sure they fall in line with the 3 Rules. A restaurant's job is to formulate its recipes to include ingredients that are highly addictive and keep you coming back. Unfortunately, most of the addictive ingredients are also ultra-processed, high-glycemic compounds that cause fat storage, as well as feed a host of metabolic diseases. They even pack these harmful ingredients in food they describe as healthy using the latest buzzwords to convince you that you're making smart choices. The last place you'd want to trust with being lean and healthy is the restaurant that is trying to get you *addicted* to extract more *profits*.

The following are some examples of common restaurant meals and what to eat to follow The 3.

Mexican food place: get a bowl with lettuce/cabbage, grilled or fresh veggies, grilled chicken, salsa. (Optional: add guacamole and/or sour cream.)

PRO TIP: Avoid shredded cheese because they usually add some sort of starch as an anticaking agent.

Flame broiler: get a chicken bowl with white meat and veggie only. Tell them *no sauce*, or they will put teriyaki sauce on it. You can add hot sauce as long as the ingredients are 3-Rule approved.

PRO TIP: If you eat out a lot, get some condiment packets that have 3 Rule–approved ingredients so that you can bring them with you.

Sushi: get sashimi salad with no dressing, use soy sauce, lemon and sesame oil instead. You can have spicy tuna hand rolls with no rice, adding avocado and veggies.

In-N-Out: burger wrapped in lettuce (instead of a bun) with veggies and mustard. (No spread or toppings.)

PRO TIP: Make Thousand Island dressing at home; it tastes the same as the In-N-Out sauce. (See recipe in the Dressings/Sauces section.)

At other restaurants, you can always get the following:

- Steak, chicken, or fish with grilled veggies. (Make sure there are no sauces or glazes.)
- A salad with all Three Rule–approved ingredients like a Cobb salad—hold any ingredients over 25 on the glycemic index, and don't ask for dressing. Just ask for olive oil and vinegar. (Beware of "vinaigrettes" because there is usually sugar added.)

7

Working Out

Everyone Wants to Be Stronger, No One Wants to Be Weaker

*"You never know what life is going to throw
at you, but you do know that being strong
will always give you an advantage."*

It's great to run, do yoga, spin, and hike, and I encourage you to be active doing what you love if that's your thing. All of that should be part of your fitness program, but it's not the complete picture. You may get strong in some areas, but you'll never be as strong in *all areas* as you would if you were to add lifting weights to your program. Everyone wants to be stronger, and for that to happen, you have to lift heavy things.

The worst is when people don't work out at all. I don't get it. I don't get how you can just wake up every day and know you're weaker than you were the day before. I don't get how you can show up for your family being physically weak.

For a husband, wife, father, or mother, to show up soft and weak and claim to love your family more than anything? You don't love them more than being lazy. You don't love them enough to put in 30 to 45 minutes, 3 to 5 days per week to give them the BEST version of you. Oh well, I guess they'll have to settle for the physically weak version. That's what they're worth to you?

I was watching a video on YouTube of an obese mother who tried to stop the stroller with her baby in it from rolling down a hill into oncoming traffic. She tripped and fell, and she was so fat and weak that she kept falling down. She literally couldn't save her helpless baby from being killed as it rolled toward traffic.

Over and over, she made pathetic attempts to get up, and each one failed. Luckily, at the last moment, a bystander who was in decent shape ran over and stopped the stroller with only moments to spare, avoiding catastrophe. This video should never have made it to YouTube because anyone who was decently fit could have easily jumped up and grabbed the stroller.

PRO TIP: You never know what life is going to throw at you, but you do know that being strong will always give you an advantage. Not just physically stronger; the mental strength that you get from lifting is huge.

LIFT or DIE.

TRAVEL WORKOUTS

"No matter what you have access to,
you can always get a workout in."

Before I travel, I check what kind of weight room the hotel has. Most big hotels have a decent gym these days. However, if the choice is between two similar hotels, I'll pick the one with the better gym. Remember, you're creating your *character*. Your character is someone who eats healthy, is disciplined, and has a positive mental attitude. You don't leave your character at home. If it's really *who* you are, then you don't break character.

No matter what you have access to, you can always get a workout in. If, for some reason, you don't have access to a gym, you can just do a bodyweight workout. Time yourself. How fast can you get 100 pushups, 100 air squats, and 100 burpee pushups? That workout is no joke. If you're trying to beat your last time, even doing the exact same workout will never become easy. When you're done—*you did it*. You got it in. You chose being *proud*.

CONSISTENCY IS KEY

"Not every workout has to be a world-destroyer."

My default setting is to push myself as much as I can every workout. Yet there are times I back off a bit, such as when I'm sick, have an injury, or I can just tell that I'm run down.

Not every workout has to be a world-destroyer. Consistency is so much more important that going all out but missing workouts or burning out because of it. However, be aware of your mindset when you're not going all out. Do you really have a legit reason, or are you just being mentally weak? When you don't feel like pushing, and you do anyway, you're practicing being *mentally strong*; if you give in, you're practicing being mentally weak.

The prospect of being mentally weak scares me. I don't think a lot of people look at it like this, but I think that if I'm mentally weak in this moment, what will prevent me from being weak in the next moment? What's different about the next moment? What thought process will I use to not give in next time?

Well, then why don't I just use that thought process this time?

Like I said, if you have a legit reason for not going all out, then do what you have to do. It's all about being consistent and keeping the routine going. For example, a coaching client of mine named Mike had dental surgery. His dentist told him not to work out for at least a week. Did he stay home? No. He still got up in the morning, showed up at the gym, and walked on the treadmill. He did not break character or his routine.

MISSING WORKOUTS IS KILLING YOUR CONFIDENCE

"The difference in the potential of all things between a person who is confident and someone who isn't is exponential."

The biggest thing that either builds up your confidence or tears it down is keeping your word to yourself. If your conscience is telling you to work out, and you've made that agreement with yourself, then each time you don't hold your word you lose *confidence*. I know a lot of people with big dreams, but if they can't even follow through with working out 30 to 45 minutes, how will they have the belief in themselves that they'll follow through in other areas? This is the biggest thing holding people back from reaching their full potential.

Would you have confidence in someone who lied to you all the time? If you don't fully trust that you'll keep your word because you've consistently proved it to yourself, then you'll never be confident. The difference in the potential of all things between a person who is confident and someone who isn't is *exponential.*

Choose Proud Over Happy

*"Perpetual happiness isn't possible, but
you can be perpetually proud."*

The biggest reason that I see for people missing their workouts is because they either sleep in or stop at home after work and sit down "just for second," then don't get back up off the couch. In these moments, they're choosing what makes them happy in the moment over being proud of themselves. It would make them proud to get up when their alarm goes off, but they would be happier if they hit the snooze and slept in.

The problem with choosing happy over proud is that happiness needs contrast, and you now owe a debt. You can't have *pleasure* without *pain,* just like you can't have light without dark or hot without cold. So, now you owe a debt that needs to be paid. It may come in the form of not feeling that edge that you do from working out. It may come in the form of guilt. It may come in the form of making it that much harder to get up with your alarm the next day. It might make your whole day feel off. Either way, just know that the debt is coming, and the universe *will* collect.

On the other hand, when you choose proud, the contrast and debt is already built in. The contrast and debt of getting up when you don't want to are overcoming the struggle. You paid the debt by feeling the pain of getting up when you didn't want to. Now you can feel proudly debt-free.

Everyone wants to be perpetually happy. The problem is that perpetual happiness isn't possible, but you can be perpetually *proud.*

Proud is a better and higher-frequency feeling than being happy. Imagine how you'd feel if you won the lottery and had a million dollars piled on your kitchen table. You'd be pretty happy. Now, imagine if you *earned* that million dollars—you'd feel so proud. If you can cycle back and forth between feeling happy versus proud, you'd choose proud every time.

What if we lived our lives by only doing what makes us proud? I urge you to choose *being proud* over happy. Finding the mindset that makes you proud doesn't get more real than with my client Lorena. This is her story, in her words:

On the night of Christmas Eve in 2019, I received a call from my sister telling me my brother-in-law had suffered a major heart attack and was in the hospital fighting for his life. He ended up passing away.

My sister went into a depression. We moved in together, and one of our mechanisms to cope with the loss and help my sister to heal was working out at OC|FIT. The workouts were intense, and for that one hour, we left our worries and sadness outside the door.

Then, in June 2024, my sister was in a severe car accident. I was devastated and scared for her. I took care of my sister during her recovery. It was the most emotionally painful situation of my life. After a week of having her home with me, I was debating whether to go back to OC|FIT and continue in the program. I was so used to having my partner in crime with me, and going without her was going to be like missing a huge part of me.

But when I was helping my sister get up the stairs, I remem-bered one of Steve's coaching calls and his message to think of working out and staying healthy as we "Get" to do this. I remembered the story he shared about his friend who had been paralyzed in a football accident and realized that I was experiencing that "Get" feeling.

I Get to work out. I Get to feel soreness. I Get to wake up. I Get to walk, while my sister was struggling to take a single step. She encouraged me to keep going in the program and working out at OC|FIT. I encouraged her to keep going in the program too (at least with the eating habits).

I ended up staying, continuing my journey. It was not easy. But I was more motivated than ever! I felt I had to work out for my sister and myself. She could not. I was able to. I Get to do this.

At times, I don't know if it was sweat or tears that were rolling down, but one thing was for sure, I was so grateful to be able to make a tough OC|FIT workout, and Steve was a strong influence in keeping my mindset healthy and seeing once again the who I was on the inside shining through to the outside.

Work On Character

*"This muscle you're developing in your mind
can and will be used in all aspects of life."*

I want you to look at working out as working on your character. Every workout, every set, every rep—even just getting up to work out is a chance to practice working on your character. It's an opportunity to build yourself into someone you're proud of. Someone whom you admire.

During every set, there comes a time when it burns. When you want to stop. But you don't. You *push through* for a few more reps. You practice *mental fortitude*. This muscle you're developing in your mind can and will be used in all aspects of life. Guess what? The days that I don't want to work out are the ones I love the most because I get the most character from those days.

DISCIPLINE VERSUS MOTIVATION

*"Relying on motivation is the same as
being controlled by my feelings."*

Do you think I'm always motivated to work out? Of course not! I have a family, multiple businesses, and I don't get much sleep. I'd say that 70 to 80 percent of the time I don't feel "motivated" to work out. Relying on motivation is the same as being controlled by my feelings.

I rely on discipline. I rely on my character and knowing who I am. I am not someone who succumbs to weakness. I *will not* accept that.

The way I feel on a particular day about working out means nothing to me. I rely on being someone I'm proud of. Someone I admire. Someone who shows up for his family, friends, and others as the best version of himself. When I feel motivated, it's a bonus, but I will never *rely* on it. *Choose discipline over motivation.*

You are capable of so much more then you think. By proving to yourself that you can do the little things like staying on your nutrition and not missing workouts, you earn the confidence that you can do the big things—this mindset shift is life-changing.

SORENESS

*"If you stay consistent with your workouts,
you'll be less sore every week."*

One of the biggest mistakes that I see beginners make is waiting until they're not sore to do their next workout. Let me tell you how it works. When you're a beginner, or if you haven't worked out for around two weeks, you can and will get extremely sore after working out. It's just because your body isn't used to it.

For example, the first time you hit legs, you may feel like you can hardly walk. You may think, "How can I keep this up for the rest of my life? This totally sucks!" So you wait until you're not sore to work legs again because you think that will help. But, nope, you waited too long and end up just as sore the next time around. So you quit working out; you decide you'd rather be weak.

Here's what you need to know. As long as you stick to the program and don't wait longer than a week to hit that same muscle group again, you will be about 70 percent less sore on your second workout. If you stay consistent, you will only be about 10 to 15 percent as sore as your first workout. It's what we call the good sore. It's the sore you crave because it lets you know you had a good workout. If you're a beginner or haven't worked out in a long time, pay your debt and suck it up for the first week. Your second week will be way different. Just stick with the program.

FEELING INTIMIDATED

"Who really cares what people think?"

A big reason a lot of people stick to the cardio equipment and stay out of the weight room is because they're afraid they'll look stupid. They think that they'll be judged for not having proper form.

First off, people aren't looking at you (unless you're doing some really dumb exercise you saw on YouTube or TikTok, like trying to do cable crossovers and burpee pushups at the same time). People are focused on themselves. Second, who really cares what people think? Everyone was a beginner at some point, and the only way to get good at something is by doing it. Just stick to the workout program that I made for you in this book.

You can go to www.stevehochman.com to watch the workout videos where I show you exactly what your form should look like. Put your headphones on and get to work.

FOCUS ON THE WORK, NOT THE RESULT

"When you become the who,
you look like the what."

PRO TIP: Don't get hyper-focused on the results. The results will come with time. The focus should be on *who* you're becoming. Choosing to work out is about who you are. Pushing through the pain of the last few reps shows who you are. Being *consistent, disciplined*, and *determined* is a reflection of who you are. The person who I am does certain things and does not do others. I look like who I am. When you become the who, you look like the what.

One of the most inspiring members of my community is Josie, Lorena's sister. Their support for each other is incredible, and a true example of connecting to a higher purpose. In her words:

I was in a car accident, which resulted in sacrum, hip, nose, and eye fractures. I was in the hospital for three days, in severe pain, unable to walk (thank God only temporarily) and unable to do everyday tasks. There were a handful of people—angels—who I can say without hesitation were pivotal in my recovery: my amazing sister Lorena, my parents, and Steve Hochman.

I had joined his nutritional challenge a couple of months before my accident, and I truly believe the learning/education on nutrition that Steve provided and the results I experienced in just a couple of months "set up/prepared" me to be able to recover more speedily after the accident. I asked my doctor and physical therapist, and they agree. In spite of the inability to attend workout sessions, I kept posting my food logs, and Steve graciously reviewed them for me. In time, I was able to return to working out alongside my sister.

Being in the program along with my sister Lorena has been amazing. I am extremely grateful that we've had each other throughout this program and this journey, which continues. We keep each other accountable, support each other, and celebrate each other's success. Just today, a coworker said I look ten years younger. I have lost about two dress sizes, and I'm back to feeling healthy and strong. Every single coach at OC|FIT is amazing and provides us with a challenging workout that sharpens us not only physically but also mentally. It's gratifying to see the physical/aesthetic results, yet the most important is to have that unwavering mindset and purpose. Enjoy the journey!

Connect to a Higher Purpose

"We are not a big enough reason."

Remember, none of this is about just you. We've already established that we will lie, bargain with, and let ourselves down. We are not a big enough reason. Connect your workouts to a *higher purpose* than yourself.

Remember this from earlier in the book: If you're a parent who convinces yourself that it's okay to be mentally weak and miss your workout, you don't have the right to tell your kids what to do for their best interests. At the very least, you really can't look them in the eye and say it with the same conviction if you aren't doing what you're supposed to do.

Tell yourself that when you choose to miss your workouts, you're choosing to hurt your kids or that being lazy is more important to you than helping your kids. Helping them by leading them by example. Kids listen to 10 percent of what we say but emulate 90 percent of what we do.

Community and Coaching

*"The best workout in the entire world
is the one you do consistently."*

One of the best ways to really make that change and become the best version of yourself is to immerse yourself into a community of others who are on the same path. As the motivational speaker Jim Rohn said, "We are the average of the five people we spend the most time with." You hang out with five losers, and you'll be the sixth.

My coaching program provides mindset, accountability, workouts, and nutrition; live weekly coaching calls for personal development; and a community of like-minded people on the path to become the person that they are proud of and admire. Everyone here is becoming the best version of themselves, and so can you. I truly know that nothing compares to having a coach in your corner. Go to www.stevehochman.com and apply for coaching today.

This whole book is about sharing what works for me. It's what has taken me from being obese, undisciplined, and weak-minded to having a six pack and an *unbreakable* mindset. The cool thing is that the same plan that worked for me has also worked for more than *1,000* personal clients, and hundreds of thousands of clients through my franchises.

When I first transformed myself from fat to shredded, I had hours of free time. I was single with no kids and few responsibilities. Quickly, that all changed, and within a year or two, I ran a seven-figure personal training studio, had a combination of more than 45 employees and private contractors, and had a wife and kids. Out of necessity, I was forced to create short, 45-minute workouts that were as effective as my 3-hour workout had been.

When you go to the gym, you'll see most people do a set, then check their phone for a few minutes. After they're all done lifting, then they do some sort of cardio. My workouts have practically *zero rest*. Because of the pace, I end up getting cardio at the same time that I'm lifting. And because of the pace, I get everything done in about 45 minutes.

Every gym is different, plus some people work out at home, and others have injuries or limitations. The following workout is what I do. You can modify it for you and what you have access to. If you need to reduce the number of sets until you work up to the full workout, go for it.

For any movements you aren't familiar with or for which you don't know the proper form, head to www.stevehochman. com for detailed videos and instruction.

Or, if you want to have custom workouts, nutrition, accountability, and personal development, head to www.stevehochman. com and apply for coaching with me. And remember, the *best workout* in the entire world is the one you *do consistently*.

WHY I DO A FIVE-DAY SPLIT

"Five days per week is my minimum."

How many days per week should you work out? I believe the magic number is five. It's called a five-day split because you split working out the different parts of your body over five days. I think that three days per week is the minimum to maintain your current fitness level. You're working out less than half the week. Four days per week is perfect for making noticeable progress. You're working out more than half the days in a week. Five days per week is my minimum.

I use five days as a benchmark because even though you can see progress with four days, it still leaves three days per week for you to fall out of your routine. Personally, I do six or seven days per week: four or five really hard workouts, and one or two lighter workouts. I work out as much for *mental strength* as I do for *physical strength*.

On Workout 5, 6, and 7, I go back and hit some of the muscle groups that I hit earlier in the week. You want to have one to three days between hitting the same muscles because when you work out, you break your muscles down; when you recover, your body repairs the damaged muscles and makes them stronger so they can handle the stress better next time. That's why you don't want to work the same exact muscles every day.

With that said, if some crazy scenario made it so I either had to work the same muscles every day for a week or nothing at all, I'd work the same muscles. Your body still makes some repairs in just one night of sleep, so there are no excuses.

WORKOUTS FOR ALL LEVELS: BEGINNER TO ADVANCED

These workouts are structured to accommodate individuals at different fitness levels and designed for people with access to a commercial gym like 24 Hour Fitness. Beginners can start with lighter weights, fewer sets, and a comfortable pace. As you progress, increase difficulty using the following methods.

These workouts have been created for busy people who have 45 minutes or less to get some!

1. Start with two sets per exercise and gradually work up to five sets.
2. Complete workouts faster, timing yourself to establish a baseline, then set a goal to beat your time.
3. Gradually increase the weight used for each exercise.

Day 1: Legs (HIIT Focus)

Warm-Up:

- Five-minute light cardio (treadmill, bike, or rowing machine).

Workout:

1. Assault Bike (or any cardio equipment): 20 calories for men/10 calories for women.
2. Weighted Walking Lunges: 20 steps.
3. Goblet Squats with Dumbbell: 15 reps.
   - ▷ Perform 2–5 rounds as a circuit.
4. Deficit Reverse Lunges: 10 reps per leg.
   - ▷ Place your front foot on a weight plate for added range of motion.
   - ▷ Perform 2–5 sets.
5. Leg Press: 15 reps.
   - ▷ Super-Set with Bodyweight Jump Squats: 15 reps.
   - ▷ Perform 2–5 rounds.
6. Seated Calf Raises: 25 reps.
   - ▷ Perform 2–5 sets.

Day 2: Chest, Shoulders, and Triceps

Warm-Up:
- Five-minute light cardio or dynamic stretches.

Workout:

1. Dumbbell Side Lateral Raises: 20 reps.
2. Dumbbell Front Raises: 10 reps (both arms simultaneously).
3. Dumbbell Shoulder Press: 15 reps.
4. Burpee Push-Ups: 20 reps.
   - ▷ Perform 2–5 rounds as a circuit.
5. Alternating Dumbbell Forward Raises (palms facing in) 12 reps per side.
6. Upright Rows with Dumbbells: 12 reps.
7. Alternating shoulder press: 20 reps total.
   - ▷ Perform 2–5 rounds as a circuit.
8. Dumbbell Chest Press: 15–20 reps.
9. Dumbbell Chest Flies: 12 reps.
10. Push-Ups: 25 reps (modify to knees if needed).
    - ▷ Perform 2–5 rounds as a circuit.
11. Triceps Extensions (Straight Bar Cable): 20 reps.
12. Skull Crushers (bar or dumbbells): 15 reps.
13. Overhead Dumbbell Triceps Extensions: 12–15 reps.
    - ▷ Perform 2–5 rounds.

Day 3: Back and Biceps

Warm-Up:
- Five-minute light cardio or band pull-aparts.

Workout:

1. TRX Reverse Flies: 15 reps.
2. TRX Face Pulls: 15 reps.
3. Dumbbell Reverse Flies: 20 reps (standing, bent over).
   - ▷ Perform 2–5 rounds as a circuit.
4. Pull-Ups: Perform until failure up to 15 reps (use assisted pull-up machine if necessary).
   - ▷ Perform 2–5 rounds.
5. Dumbbell Rows: 15 reps per side.
   - ▷ Perform 2–5 sets.
6. Straight Arm Cable Pushdowns: 20 reps.
7. EZ Bar Curls: 12 reps, followed by a drop set (10–12 additional reps with lighter weight).
   - ▷ Perform 2–5 rounds as a circuit.
8. Machine Preacher Curls: 12–15 reps.
9. Alternating Dumbbell Hammer Curls: 12 reps per side.
10. Double Dumbbell Hammer Curls: 12 reps (both arms simultaneously).
    - ▷ Perform 2–5 rounds as a circuit.

Day 4: Deadlift, Abs, and Lower Back (HIIT)

Warm-Up:
- Five-minute light cardio or dynamic stretches.

Workout:

1. Hyperextensions: 15 reps (bodyweight or with a weight plate).
2. Dumbbell or Bar Romanian Dead Lifts (RDL): 15 reps.
3. Kettlebell Swings: 15 reps.
4. Burpee Push-Ups: 20 reps.
   ▷ Perform 2–5 rounds as a circuit.
5. Ball Crunches: 30 reps.
6. Hanging Leg Raises: 20 reps (use ab straps or Roman chair if necessary).
7. Plank Bridge: Hold for 1 minute.
   ▷ Perform 2–5 rounds as a circuit.
8. Side Plank (each side): 30 seconds per side.
   ▷ Perform 2–5 sets.

Day 5: Full-Body Compound Movements

Warm-Up:
- Five-minute light cardio or dynamic stretches.

Workout:

1. Triple Burpee Push-Ups: 10 reps (3 push-ups per rep).
2. Hammer Curls: 15 reps.
3. Hammer Curl Presses: 15 reps.
4. Side Lateral Raises: 15 reps.
   - ▷ Perform 2–5 rounds as a circuit.
5. Pull-Ups: Perform until failure (target 12–15 reps).
6. Dumbbell Rows: 15 reps per side.
7. Upright Rows with Dumbbells: 15 reps.
8. Dumbbell Squat Press: 15 reps.
   - ▷ Perform 2–5 rounds as a circuit.

Progression Tips:

- **Beginners:** Start with 2 sets, use light weights, and focus on proper form.
- **Intermediate:** Perform 3–4 sets, increase weight moderately, and aim to maintain a steady pace.
- **Advanced:** Perform 5 sets, use heavy weights, and time yourself to push intensity.

You're Not Fully Living If You're Not Lifting

Stefanie is a perfect example of the power of The 3 combined with lifting weights. In her words:

For most of my life, I was naturally thin, able to eat whatever I wanted without a second thought. That changed in my 30s. Fresh out of grad school, I committed to making my health a priority, diving into exercise and what I thought was "healthy" eating. I started by cutting calories, convinced that consuming less would yield results. But despite working out consistently—sometimes pushing through intense HIIT workouts followed by three-mile runs six days a week—I wasn't seeing the definition or weight loss I expected. Frustrated and confused, I decided it was time to consult an expert.

That's when I met Steve, whose nutritional approach, later known as The 3, completely reshaped my perspective. Now, full disclosure before I go on: Steve and I are happily married and have been together for about nine years! When we first met, though, he was my nutrition coach and the owner of OC|FIT, the program I joined. Steve introduced me to concepts I'd never considered, like the glycemic index. Rather than focusing only on calories, he showed me that what I ate mattered far more than how much. I left that first meeting feeling inspired and ready to try a whole new approach to food.

After a tough, two-week detox from all the hidden, addictive, high-glycemic foods I'd been eating, I began noticing real changes. I felt more energized, my workout endurance improved, and I finally began seeing the muscle definition I'd been striving for. This wasn't just a diet—it was a sustainable, balanced way of eating that felt liberating rather than restrictive.

The impact didn't stop with me. As a mom, I want my four-year-old son to have a strong, healthy foundation, and I've adapted a kid-friendly version of The 3 for him, as well. Helping him grow up strong and healthy by adopting The 3 has been an incredibly rewarding experience. We've taught him about the downsides of excess sugar and bad carbs, and he's already developing a healthy relationship with food and understands the benefits of choosing real, nourishing options over sugary treats. His teachers have even told me that before he accepts a treat, he'll ask if it contains "real" sugar. As a mom, that's a proud win!

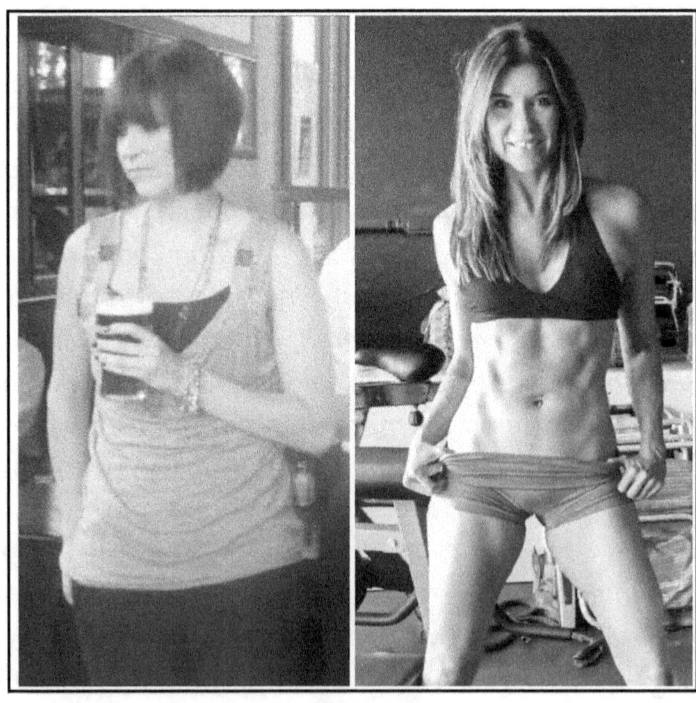

To recap:

- Lifting weights is ESSENTIAL for improving your overall strength; other exercises without lifting WON'T CUT IT.
- Strength training builds physical and mental resilience
- Regular workouts are more beneficial than the occasional, intense session; discipline is WAY more sustainable motivation.
- Keep your word to yourself and do the workouts—that's the key to gaining confidence and becoming the WHO you want to be.
- Do the things that make you proud—always choose PROUD over happy.
- A five-day split is the benchmark for lifting—you'll make great progress and still give your body plenty of recovery time.

8
Let's Wrap This Up

No matter what your life is like, it is exponentially enhanced by being lean, fit, and proud of *who* you are. I'm going to share two more stories with you that I think illustrate this perfectly.

There's a powerful universal law called the law of exposure. If you're exposed to something long enough, you adopt it.

My wife and I hired a nanny named Krystal to help us with our three-year-old. She'd struggled with her weight her whole life. Krystal saw me and my wife make all our food day after day. I don't usually approach people who I'm around a lot or who work for me about nutrition unless they ask me. Some people just aren't ready, and I don't want it to get awkward. But she kept asking me questions like, "Why do you eat this?" "Why do you make it that way?" "Why don't you eat that?" Each time, I'd answer her, and slowly I taught her The 3. I also let her try the foods I was making, and she couldn't believe meals that get you super lean could taste this good.

She started incorporating The 3 Monday through Friday when she was at our house. It was partly because she loved the food, and partly because she was embarrassed to eat badly in front us. In her own words:

When I first started working for the Hochman family, I was nearly 200 pounds. As time went on, I started changing my

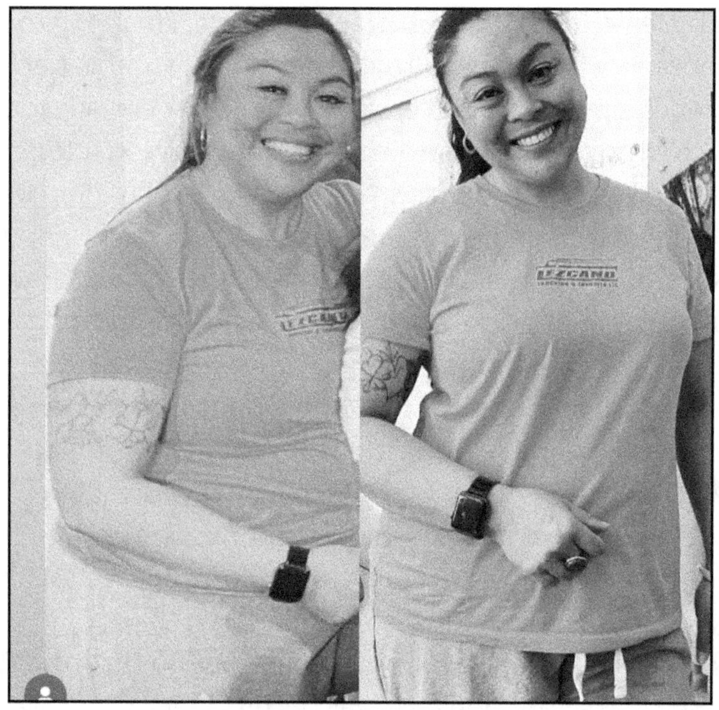

The people you surround yourself with and are exposed to matters. One of the best things you can do to make a positive change is to immerse yourself into a community of people who are living how you want to live and change yourself through the law of exposure.

I met a girl named Gina, who was prediabetic. This meant that if she didn't make a major change, she was going to have *full-blown* diabetes and require insulin. She told me she was so terrified because many of her family members had diabetes, and she'd seen them have parts of their body amputated because of it.

As a mom, she wanted to end this family cycle and give her kids the life they deserve. We got started on my coaching program that day. When I got her first food log, I was pretty shocked. It was tacos from Taco Bell, a Slurpee from 7-Eleven, and cookies after dinner. I called and said, "Hey Gina, I just read your food log and I'm really surprised by what I'm seeing here. You told me you're scared to death of your kids experiencing the same pain that you are, just like your parents did to you. But your food log makes it look like you haven't really found your higher purpose, and I can't force you to care more about your health." She got upset and said maybe she's not ready for this program.

Ready? Are you ready for diabetes? Ready to have your limbs amputated? Ready to pass your *pain* and *unhealthy habits* on to your kids? I refunded her and that was that.

PRO TIP: The sad reality is that there have to be losers in this world for there to be winners. Just like you can't have light without darkness or pleasure without pain, you can't have winners without losers. As a parent, passing pain on to your kids is something I can never understand. Unfortunately, on the path she's chosen, Gina will probably realize this when it's too late. Don't let the fact that Gina volunteered to be one of the losers go to waste. Let's learn from her and never be like Gina.

This book is a vehicle for you to become the best version of yourself. There is no way to get to that version while putting poison in your body, breaking character, and not being in alignment with your conscience.

However, you need to have the drive. I can't make you want it. That drive is in you. It's called your conscience. It's that voice or feeling pulling you in a direction. That "feeling" of not being satisfied. That "voice" that says you were meant for more, like the one I heard when I was homeless, sleeping on the floor, and the cigarette ash was about to fall on my face.

Even though your conscience is guiding you, many people are so used to either ignoring it or telling themselves so many lies and stories that they can barely hear it. Just like building muscle on your body, with complete self-honesty and a desire to become the best version of yourself, over time you can increase the volume of the voice of your conscience. But the choice is yours.

The path to your highest version of self isn't an easy path, and you don't want it to be. Personal development isn't born out of easy. The only easy part is the *choice*. Because you know in your heart that that is what your conscience is calling you to do.

I can't stress enough the importance of being aligned with your conscience. It's the ONLY way to truly find peace. I can't fathom how someone can go through their whole life without experiencing this.

RECAP OF THE 3

FIRST, connect your health and fitness goals to:

1. A higher purpose than yourself
2. Your character and who *you* are

Mindset is the key. I can give you all the "information," but if you don't have the discipline and higher purpose connection to apply as part of your daily habits, it's useless. You need to habitually create the best version of yourself and become the person you admire.

Rule 1—Keep all ingredients you eat below 25 on the glycemic index (GI). To do this, you must Google or ask ChatGPT the GI of all food and all ingredients that you eat until you become familiar with them.

Rule 2—We define a "carb" as any food or ingredient over 25 on the GI. Don't combine carbs and more than 5 grams of fat together in the same meal.

Rule 3—Use "Strategic Carb Timing." Have carbs once daily and under five grams of fat with this meal. Your carbs will be a combo of glucose like fruit or honey, and starch like potatoes, rice, or oatmeal. For the protein, I use grass-fed whey protein or egg whites made with no oil.

Accelerator #1—Drink at least half a gallon of the Magic Fat-Shred Drink per day. A lot of times when you feel hungry, you're really just thirsty. This is because the same part of your brain that sends signals when you're hungry is the same part of the brain that tells us we are thirsty. Besides a ton of health benefits, staying hydrated greatly reduces your cravings for food.

Here's the recipe one more time for the **Magic Fat-Shred Drink**. I use, and recommend, a 64oz (.5 gallon) Hydro Flask. Adjust portions for smaller containers.

- A dash of cayenne pepper (As much as you like so it gives you a little kick, but still tastes amazing)
- ¼ cup apple cider vinegar (You can use more if you like, just be careful because too much and it will dominate the drink.)
- One serving flavored low sodium sugar-free electrolytes, sweetened with stevia. (I use a brand called Ultima because it has 55 mg, it's sweetened with stevia, and tastes amazing.)
- Water (Fill the rest of the Hydro Flask with water.)

Accelerator #2—Magic 36-Hour Fast. Shred fat and increase your insulin sensitivity by doing a 36-hour fast every week to two weeks.

Be sure to burn off as much glycogen as possible by working out and doing a couple hours of steady state cardio on the day you don't eat, and the next day before you break your fast.

Accelerator #3—Intermittent fasting four to seven days per week. Don't eat for 16 hours, then have all your meals in an 8-hour eating window.

The benefit is more fat burning because of fasted workouts and increased insulin sensitivity. Be sure to drink one gallon of the Magic Fat-Shred Drink during your fasting window. Also, it's very important to break your fast with your Strategic Carb Timing (SCT) meal (carbs and protein). No fat in this meal.

And don't worry, it's not rocket science. This meal can be very simple. This is my favorite SCT meal:

- 1 cup fat-free Greek yogurt
- 1 scoop whey protein
- 1 cup berries
- 2 red potatoes on the side

If you've absorbed the information in this book, you have the nutrition knowledge that 95 percent of the population does not. You are now ready to enhance every aspect of your life through nutrition, fitness, and mindset.

With that said, I know that so many people benefit exponentially by having someone coach them and hold them accountable. Having a mentor whom they can access to help them adopt a new, unbreakable mindset will unlock the door to their highest self—the self that fully aligns with their conscience.

I've coached and helped thousands of people. My system works every time, and it's the reason I've been put on this earth. If you'd like me to help you, apply for coaching with me at www.stevehochman.com.

***The **Bonus Accelerator** I want to share with you in this book is Food Journaling. This is a phrase that I want you to burn in your mind: "Before you *bite it, write it.*" Just the very act of writing down what you eat *before* you eat it will help you make choices that align with your conscience. Keeping a food log is something all my personal clients do, so that I can review them and make sure they're on the right track.

These are examples of food logs that follow The 3 perfectly. You can use these as a starting place for yourself and write them out at home, or follow the link at the end to download a food log template from me.

Day One

6:00 a.m.—Breakfast
- **Black coffee** (GI 0)
- **Splash of unsweetened almond milk** (GI 0–5, minimal amount)
- **Squirt of liquid stevia** (GI 0)
- **4 eggs** (GI 0)
- **2 tbsp Rao's Marinara Sauce** (GI ~20)
- **1 tbsp Primal Kitchen Buffalo Ranch** (GI 2–5)
- **1 oz 4505 Sea Salt Pork Rinds** (GI 0)

9:00 a.m.—Snack
- **1 cup cottage cheese** (GI ~10)

12:00 p.m.—Lunch
- **6 oz flank steak, seasoned with sea salt** (GI 0)
- **1 cup air-fried broccoli** (GI 15)

3:00 p.m.—Snack
- **1 Chomps Beef Stick** (GI 0)

6:00 p.m.—Dinner
- **6 oz baked salmon** (GI 0)
- **1 cup steamed asparagus** (GI 15)

9:00 p.m.—Dessert
- **Chocolate Lava Cake** (GI each ingredient is below 25)

Day Two

8:00 a.m.—Breakfast
- **3 whole eggs** (GI 0)
- **¼ avocado** (GI 15)
- **1 cup sautéed spinach in olive oil** (GI 0)
- **Black coffee or tea (unsweetened)** (GI 0)

11:00 a.m.—Snack
- **3 slices rolled turkey with organic mustard** (GI 0)
- **2 celery sticks** (GI 0)
- **1 tbsp organic peanut butter** (GI ~20, optional)

2:00 p.m.—Lunch
- **6 oz grilled chicken breast** (GI 0)
- **1 cup cauliflower mash** (garlic, rosemary) (GI 15)
- **1 cup steamed broccoli** (GI 15)
- **2 tbsp ranch dressing** (Side Dish brand) (GI 5)

3:00 p.m. Workout
5:00 p.m.—SCT
- **1 cup fat-free Greek yogurt** (GI 11)
- **¼ cup blueberries** (GI 53)
- **1 scoop whey protein powder** (unsweetened) (GI 0)
- **1 tbsp beetroot powder** (GI 61–85)

8:00 p.m.—Dinner
- **6 oz baked salmon** (GI 0)
- **1 cup steamed asparagus with lemon** (GI 15)
- **1 cup side salad (mixed greens) with olive oil and balsamic vinegar** (GI 0)

Day Three

5:00 a.m.—Early Breakfast
- **Black coffee** (GI 0)
- **Splash of unsweetened almond milk** (GI 5)
- **1 tbsp liquid stevia** (GI 0)
- **4 scrambled eggs** (GI 0)
- **2 tbsp salsa (no added sugar)** (GI ~15)
- **1 oz pork rinds** (GI 0)

8:00 a.m.—Breakfast
- **1 cup non-fat Greek yogurt** (GI 11)
- **1 scoop vanilla whey protein powder** (unsweetened) (GI 0)
- **¼ cup chopped walnuts** (GI 15)
- **Dash of cinnamon** (GI 0)

11:00 a.m.—Snack
- **Air-fried bell peppers** (GI 15)

2:00 p.m.—Lunch
- **6 oz grilled chicken breast, seasoned with sea salt** (GI 0)
- **1 cup air-fried zucchini** (GI 15)
- **1 cup mixed green salad with olive oil and balsamic vinegar** (GI 0)

4 p.m. Workout
5:00 p.m.—SCT
- **1 cup fat-free Greek yogurt** (GI 11)
- **¼ cup blueberries** (GI 40–53)
- **1 scoop chocolate whey protein powder** (unsweetened) (GI 0)
- **1 tbsp beetroot powder** (GI 61–85)

8:00 p.m.—Dinner
- **6 oz baked salmon with lemon juice** (GI 0)
- **1 cup steamed broccoli** (GI 15)
- **1 cup side salad (cucumber, spinach, and red onion) with olive oil and vinegar** (GI 0)

Download your free food log template
here: www.stevehochman.com

www.ingramcontent.com/pod-product-compliance
Lightning Source LLC
Chambersburg PA
CBHW071615030726
47598CB00001B/285